Brain Mapping and Working

Brain Mapping and Working

Edited by **Noah Martin**

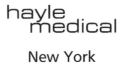

New York

Published by Hayle Medical,
30 West, 37th Street, Suite 612,
New York, NY 10018, USA
www.haylemedical.com

Brain Mapping and Working
Edited by Noah Martin

International Standard Book Number: 978-1-63241-063-4 (Hardback)

Contents

Preface

Functional brain mapping has acquired significant influence on academic and clinical practice and a large amount of grants are being issued to this branch of neuroscience to boost experimental and practical implementations, and to uncover the mysteries in this field. The most successful approach to unlock the mysteries of the brain, as said by Jay Ingram, is to bring together an interdisciplinary network of scientists and clinicians to encourage an interchange of ideas. This method of exchange is the main focus of this book. Some of the main chapters included in this book are cross modal influence of odor hedonics on facial attractiveness: behavioural and fMRI measures, optimized signal separation for 3D-polarized light imaging, causal relationships and network parameters in effective brain connectivity, and mapping of angiogenesis by magnetic resonance imaging.

After months of intensive research and writing, this book is the end result of all who devoted their time and efforts in the initiation and progress of this book. It will surely be a source of reference in enhancing the required knowledge of the new developments in the area. During the course of developing this book, certain measures such as accuracy, authenticity and research focused analytical studies were given preference in order to produce a comprehensive book in the area of study.

This book would not have been possible without the efforts of the authors and the publisher. I extend my sincere thanks to them. Secondly, I express my gratitude to my family and well-wishers. And most importantly, I thank my students for constantly expressing their willingness and curiosity in enhancing their knowledge in the field, which encourages me to take up further research projects for the advancement of the area.

Editor

Experimental and Clinical Applications of Functional Neuroimaging

The Crossmodal Influence of Odor Hedonics on Facial Attractiveness: Behavioural and fMRI Measures

Francis McGlone, Robert A. Österbauer,
Luisa M. Demattè and Charles Spence

Additional information is available at the end of the chapter

1. Introduction

Facial attractiveness is a highly relevant social cue, readily assessed by human observers. Facial attractiveness significantly impact on success in both work and social environments [1, 2]. Taking a Darwinian perspective, Perrett at al. [3] have argued that the physical structure of beautiful faces – as judged by others – provide salient signals of mate value that motivate behavior in others. Several general features have been shown to contribute to the perceived attractiveness of a face, including both facial symmetry and the extent to which an individual face conforms to an average prototype [4, 5, 6]. Additionally, faces displaying various emotional expressions (e.g., joy, anger, etc.) have been used to investigate the brain regions involved in the coding of affect [7, 8, 9, 10, 11], such as the orbitofrontal cortex (OFC), the insular cortex, and the amygdala.

At both an explicit and implicit level, humans through the ages have devised means by which to enhance facial attractiveness (a multibillion dollar cosmetic industry attests to this fact). An equally lucrative fragrance industry exploits the hedonic primacy of odors in the human brain, yet it remains unclear whether the presence of odors can modulate the perceived attractiveness of faces.

A pioneering positron emission tomography (PET) study by Nakamura and colleagues [12] demonstrated that activity in left frontal brain regions correlates with perceived facial attractiveness in humans. Furthermore, functional magnetic resonance imaging (fMRI) has been used to show that the viewing of attractive female faces by male participants activates reward circuitry in the brain, in particular, the nucleus accumbens and the OFC [13, 14].

A recent study investigated the neural circuitry involved in the perception of facial attractiveness more directly by presenting participants with faces of varying attractiveness, while they performed a gender discrimination task [15]. Correlation analysis with ratings of attractiveness for the presented faces revealed a region in the medial orbitofrontal cortex (OFC) that responded specifically to facial attractiveness.

Physical attractiveness is not, however, solely dependent upon the visual aspects of appearance, but is often modulated by other sensory cues. For example, a person's voice has been shown to influence a speaker's perceived attractiveness [16, 17]. Similarly, a person's body odor also influences their perceived attractiveness [18]. The notion that odors can exert an influence over the perception of facial characteristics is also supported by the observation that the perceived masculinity/femininity of faces may be modulated by the presence of human sex hormone-like chemicals [19]. Additionally, the presence of a malodor can negatively influence the perceived attractiveness of male faces as rated by female observers in a psychophysical judgment task [20].

Only a few neuroimaging experiments have simultaneously presented odors and faces to participants, but none have directly assessed the impact of odor valence on facial attractiveness. For example, an fMRI study conducted by Gottfried and colleagues [21] paired faces with either a pleasant, unpleasant, or neutral odor, in an associative learning paradigm. Their results suggest that the brain regions involved in the processing of positive and negative affect, such as OFC, nucleus accumbens, and amygdala, are engaged during the appetitive and aversive learning process. Additionally, those brain areas previously found to participate in low-level odor processing, such as the piriform cortex and the caudal OFC, were also found to play an active role in the transfer of affective value between the olfactory and visual modalities. However, since no measure of the attractiveness of the faces was obtained, it remains unclear whether odor valence actually influenced the participants' perception of the faces.

Finally, it could be argued that odors do not necessarily modulate facial attractiveness *per se*, but rather other affective components of interpersonal perception such as, for example, perceived sympathy [22]. Alternatively, however, the presentation of the odor could also induce a general change in a person's mood (or emotional state) that might also be expected to alter facial attractiveness. Indeed, the psychological and physiological literature published to date supports the view that visual stimuli can influence olfactory perception while olfactory cues rarely influence visual perception [23, 24, 25, 26]. It thus appears reasonable to assume that the simultaneous presentation of an odor will not change the visual characteristics of a face as such, but rather will primarily just changes people's affective reaction to it.

The main aim of the present study was therefore to investigate, both behaviorally and using fMRI, whether olfactory cues can modulate visual judgments of facial attractiveness. In particular, we investigated whether olfactory cues of differing hedonic value (i.e., pleasant vs. unpleasant) enhance and/or reduce the perceived attractiveness of male faces to female participants. Additionally, we selected an artificial body odor and a common male fragrance as the olfactory stimuli for their ecological relevance when paired with human faces. We hypothesized that the OFC, in particular, would show differential responses depending on the perceived attractiveness of the stimuli presented, since this brain region is activated by pleasant / unpleasant smells [27, 28, 29, 21, 30], and is also known to encode facial attractiveness [31, 15].

2. Material and methods

2.1. Participants

Twenty-one healthy right-handed female volunteers participated in this study (mean age 23 years, age range 19-29 years). All of the participants were non-smoking, had no history of nasal dysfunction or allergies to odors and each gave written informed consent after having received the written instructions concerning the study. Three participants had to be removed from the data analysis because of excessive head motion during the brain scanning session, and the data from two participants were discarded because they were unable to detect the presence versus absence of the odors at above chance levels (44% and 53% correct, respectively). Consequently, the data analysis at the group level included a total of 16 datasets. The study was approved by the Central Oxford Research Ethics Committee (C99.179).

2.2. Stimuli and task

Two odorants were used in this study, an artificial body odor (Thiol compound) and a popular male fragrance. The odors were diluted in 30ml of dipropylene glycol at concentrations of 0.0033% for the body odor and 0.5% for the male fragrance. The olfactory stimuli were delivered with a custom-built, computer-controlled olfactometer at a flow rate of 4 liters/ second, through Teflon tubes placed directly under the participant's nose. The participants were asked to breathe normally through their nose and to refrain from making any unduly strong sniffing movements. Clean medical air was delivered continuously through the olfactometer except during the delivery of the olfactory stimuli.

Twenty male faces taken from the standardized database developed by Perrett and his colleagues [3] were used as the visual stimuli. These faces have previously been rated for attractiveness on a 5-point rating scale. We used a subset of these faces, consisting of the 10 faces with the highest attractiveness ratings and the 10 faces with the lowest attractiveness ratings. Full screen color images of the faces were generated using a video projector located outside the scanner room and projected onto a translucent screen placed directly outside the bore of the magnet. A mirror fixed on the head coil allowed the participants to view the screen while lying in the scanner.

Each of the 20 faces was presented three times, once together with each of the two odors and once in the absence of any odor, resulting in the three conditions 'face-pleasant odor', 'face-unpleasant odor' and 'face-no odor'. Additionally, each odor was presented 10 times in the absence of any visual stimulus, resulting in a total of 80 trials being presented to each participant. The order of trials was randomized for each participant, with the sole constraint that the same face was never presented consecutively.

At the beginning of each trial, the participants were visually cued by the presentation of a fixation cross to breathe in and detect the presence or absence of an odor which was delivered for 2500ms following the onset of the visual cue (Figure 1). The faces were presented for 1000ms starting 1500ms after the onset of the odor stimuli. This lag between visual and olfactory stimuli was chosen on the basis of the results of a pilot study which had established that participants perceived the onset of both stimuli as concurrent when presented at this temporal delay.

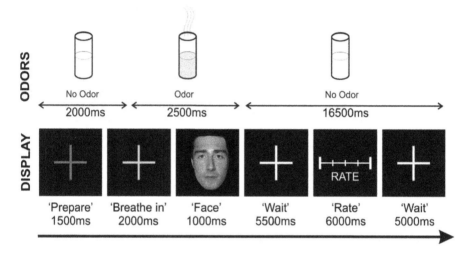

Figure 1. Participants were cued visually with a fixation cross that changed color from red to green to breathe-in and detect the presence or absence of an odor. In the trials where a face was presented, it was shown for 1000ms, beginning 2000ms after the cue to breathe in. After a rest period of 5500ms, the participants had to rate the attractiveness of the face on a 5-point rating scale. When odors were presented in the same trial, odor stimulation started 500ms after the onset of the cue to breathe-in and lasted for 2500ms, terminating together with the face. When odors were presented without a face, the cue to breathe in was displayed for 3000ms and the participants had simply to rate the pleasantness of the odor.

Following the presentation of the face, the participants rated its attractiveness on a rating scale ranging from 1='very unattractive' to 5='very attractive' with 3 as the neutral point. For the odor only trials, the participants had to rate the pleasantness of the odor on a similar scale ranging from 1='very unpleasant' to 5='very pleasant'. Behavioral measures relating to odor detection as well as the ratings were collected using a custom build button-box. The E-Prime software [32] was used to control stimulus presentation and to collect responses from the participants.

2.3. Data acquisition and analysis

Both functional and structural MRI images were acquired using a 3T Sonata Siemens scanner fitted with an 8-channel head coil (Siemens Medical Solutions, Erlangen, Germany) based at the University of Oxford Centre for Clinical Magnetic Resonance Research (OCMR). For the functional data series, a total of 1120 T2* weighted echo-planar imaging (EPI) volumes were taken over a time period of 28 min.

Each volume consisted of 27 continuous oblique (tilted approximately 20° upward from the anterior to posterior commissure line, so as to be aligned with the temporal lobes) slices of 3mm thickness with an in-plane resolution of 3×3mm. These imaging parameters allowed us to image the ventral two thirds of the brain until approximately Z-coordinate of +50 of the Montreal Neurological Institute (MNI) 152 standard brain space, to include all primary and secondary olfactory areas in the temporal lobes and OFC, as well as the visual cortex. Other imaging parameters were: TR=1.5s, 64x64 matrix, FOV 192×192 mm, TE=30ms and, flip angle = 90°.

After acquisition of the functional volumes, a B_0 field map was acquired using a combined symmetric and asymmetric spin echo sequence. For registration into standard anatomical space, a single whole brain EPI volume (50 slices, TR=5s, other imaging parameters as above) as well as a high-resolution, whole-brain T1 weighted morphological scan (inversion-recovery fast gradient echo, 1 mm slice thickness, 1mm×1mm in-plane resolution) was acquired after the experimental paradigm had been completed.

Statistical image analysis of the functional dataset was carried out using the FMRIB Expert Analysis Tool (FEAT; www.fmrib.ox.ac.uk/fsl). The following pre-processing was applied: motion correction using MCFLIRT [33]; spatial smoothing using a Gaussian kernel of FWHM 5mm; mean-based intensity normalization of all volumes by the same factor; non-linear high-pass temporal filtering (Gaussian-weighted LSF straight line fitting, sigma=25s). A general linear model using the conditions Face-No odor/Face-Body odor/Face-Fragrance/Body odor/Fragrance as explanatory variables was fitted to the time course at each voxel. Statistical analysis for each experimental run was carried out using FMRIB's Improved Linear Model (FILM) with local autocorrelation correction [34].

For group analysis, the individual results were registered both to high-resolution anatomical MR images and to the Montreal Neurological Institute (MNI) 152 standard image. Registration to high resolution and standard images was carried out using FMRIB's Linear Image Registration Tool (FLIRT) [33]. Mixed-effects (often referred to as 'random-effects') group analysis was carried out using FMRIB's Local Analysis of Mixed Effects (FLAME) software [35] with a cluster threshold of Z>2.0 and a cluster significance threshold of p=.05 (corrected for multiple comparisons) [36, 37, 38].

3. Results

3.1. Behavioral

Comparison of the pleasantness ratings when the two odors were presented in isolation confirmed that the body odor was indeed perceived as significantly [$t(15) = 8.04$; $p < .001$] less pleasant ($M = 1.78$; $SEM = 0.14$) than the fragrance ($M = 3.68$; $SEM = 0.22$), as expected. The rating data for facial attractiveness were analyzed using a repeated-measures analysis of variance (ANOVA) with the factors of facial attractiveness (low vs. high) and odor condition (pleasant, unpleasant, or odorless). As expected, the results revealed a significant main effect of facial attractiveness, [$F(1,15) = 138.23$, $p < .001$], with participants judging the pre-selected attractive faces as being more attractive ($M = 3.56$; $SEM = 0.11$) than those faces pre-selected to be less attractive ($M = 2.15$; $SEM = 0.1$). Crucially, the main effect of odors on ratings of facial attractiveness was also significant [$F(2,14)= 9.17$, $p < .01$], demonstrating that the odors affected the perceived attractiveness of the male faces to the female participants. Post-hoc comparisons (Bonferroni corrected) of the 3 odor conditions revealed that participants rated the same faces as being significantly less attractive when presented together with the unpleasant body odor ($M = 2.60$; $SEM = 0.09$) than when presented together with the pleasant odor ($M = 2.99$; $SEM = 0.11$; $p < .01$), or in the absence of any odor ($M = 2.97$; $SEM = 0.1$; $p < .01$; see Figure 2). The analysis of this behavioral data revealed no significant difference in mean facial attractiveness ratings between the pleasant versus odorless conditions, nor any interaction between facial attractiveness and odor pleasantness [$F(2,14) < 1$; $n.s.$].

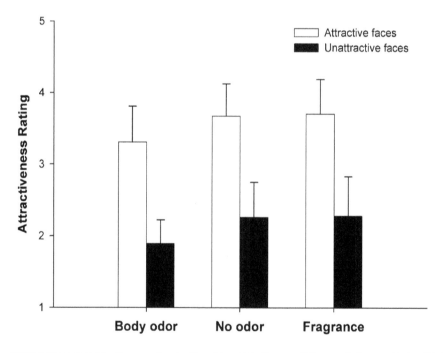

Figure 2. The average attractiveness ratings (n=16 participants) for the same 10 faces a-priori assumed to be of high attractiveness compared to the 10 low attractiveness faces are shown when either presented with an unpleasant body odor, a pleasant fragrance, or in the absence of any specific odor. The difference in ratings between the attractive and unattractive faces was significant (paired t-test, p <.05) in each odor group. Additionally, faces presented together with the body odor were rated as significantly less attractive than those presented with the fragrance or those presented in the absence of any odor (paired t-test, p <.05) for both high and low attractive faces.

3.2. Neuroimaging data

3.2.1. Odor valence

We first investigated those brain regions involved in encoding odor valence (pleasant vs. unpleasant) in the absence of any visual stimuli (i.e., faces). For this purpose, we computed two contrasts between the unimodal odor presentations, which were [Fragrance > Body odor] and [Body odor > Fragrance]. Results from the first contrasts showed several regions within the OFC to be more strongly activated by the pleasant fragrance as compared to the unpleasant odor (see Figure 3). These were located bilaterally in the medial OFC along the olfactory sulcus ($x/y/z$ = 12/44/-18; z-score = 2.62 and $x/y/z$ = -14/44/-14; z-score = 2.55), and in the lateral OFC in the right hemisphere only ($x/y/z$ = 22/50/-8; z-score = 2.63). Additionally, a small cluster was detected in the right inferior frontal gyrus pars triangularis ($x/y/z$ = 32/34/2; z-score = 2.36).

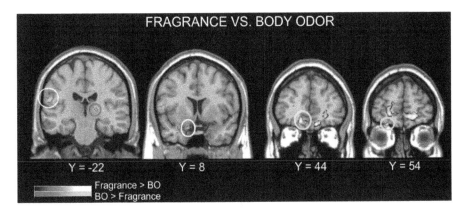

Figure 3. Group results (n=16 participants) for brain regions showing differences in brain activation relating to the pleasantness of the odors are shown on coronal slices at different y-coordinates in the canonical MNI 152 space. The contrast [Fragrance > BO] is rendered in orange/yellow and the contrast [BO > Fragrance] is rendered in blue. The unpleasant BO elicited stronger responses in the supramarginal gyrus (yellow), thalamus (red), piriform cortex (white), and lateral OFC (green). In contrast, the pleasant fragrance caused stronger activation primarily in medial OFC (turquoise). The right side of each slice corresponds to the right side of the brain.

Conversely, within the OFC, the unpleasant odor activated more strongly only in the left lateral orbital gyrus ($x/y/z$ = -24/54/-18; z-score = 2.51). However, activation was stronger in the primary sensory olfactory areas in the piriform cortex/amygdaloid area bilaterally ($x/y/z$ = 20/10/-26; z-score = 2.13 and $x/y/z$ = -16/6/22; z-score = 2.28) and in the frontal operculum ($x/y/z$ = 58/0/10; z-score = 2.13 and $x/y/z$ = -54/8/8; z-score = 2.33). Activation differences were also detected bilaterally in the supramarginal gyrus ($x/y/z$ = 58/-20/16; z-score = 2.27 and $x/y/z$ = -56/-22/22; z-score = 2.52) and in the right thalamus ($x/y/z$ = 18/-22/6; z-score = 2.30).

3.2.2. Facial attractiveness

In order to highlight those brain areas involved in encoding the attractiveness of the face stimuli independently of odors, we compared the responses to faces with high vs. low attractiveness. For these contrasts, no distinction was made between the various odor conditions (Fragrance, Body odor and clean air), which were grouped together. The results revealed that irrespective of the odor condition, the presentation of the more attractive faces led to increased BOLD signal amplitude in the medial OFC in both hemispheres ($x/y/z$ = 4/36/-8; z-score = 2.60 and $x/y/z$ = -2/36/-4; z-score = 2.96, see Figure 4). Two other brain regions also showed stronger activation in response to the more attractive faces, namely the left nucleus accumbens ($x/y/z$ = -6/8/-18; z-score = 2.93) and the hypothalamus ($x/y/z$ = 0/-6/-18; z-score = 2.69). Conversely, the presentation of the unattractive faces resulted in stronger activation bilaterally in the amygdala ($x/y/z$ = 22/0/-12; z-score = 2.19 and $x/y/z$ = -22/-4/-14; z-score = 2.45) as well as in the right pallidum ($x/y/z$ = 26/-10/-6; z-score = 2.99). Interestingly, the unattractive faces also elicited stronger activation in visual areas in the left inferior occipital gyrus ($x/y/z$ = -16/-96/-8; z-score = 2.61).

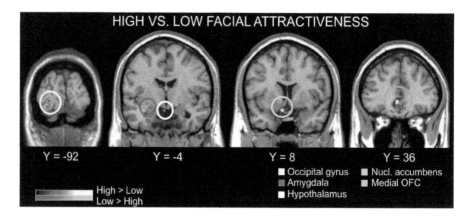

Figure 4. Group results (n=16 participants) for brain regions showing differences in brain activation relating to the attractiveness of the faces (high vs. low) are shown on coronal slices at different y-coordinates in the canonical MNI 152 space. The contrast [High > Low] is rendered in orange/yellow and the contrast [Low > High] is rendered in blue. Attractive faces preferentially engaged the medial OFC, whereas the less attractive faces led to stronger activation in the amygdala. The right side of each slice corresponds to the right side of the brain.

3.2.3. Odor-face interactions

The primary interest of the present study was to address the question of whether or not odor hedonics would influence the perceived or implicit attractiveness of male faces to female participants. The behavioral results confirmed that the same set of faces was rated as being significantly more attractive when accompanied by the pleasant odor as compared to the unpleasant odor. We were specifically interested in the brain regions associated with this effect and therefore contrasted those trials in which the faces were presented with the pleasant male fragrance to those where the same faces were presented with the unpleasant body odor. Similar to the unisensory effects of pleasant vs. unpleasant odors and attractive vs. unattractive faces, the face stimuli caused significantly stronger activation in the medial ($x/y/z$ = -6/44/-24; z-

score = 2.64) and lateral (*x/y/z* = -38/54/-16; *z-score* = 2.93) OFC as well as in the ventral striatum (*x/y/z* = -2/12/-16; *z-score* = 2.63), when they were presented together with the pleasant odor (see Figure 5). A further analysis of the percentage BOLD signal change in the peak activated voxels in the left OFC (see Figure 6) revealed positive signal changes only when faces were presented with the fragrance or in the absence of odors. The responses in these regions to all other stimuli were either close to zero or slightly negative.

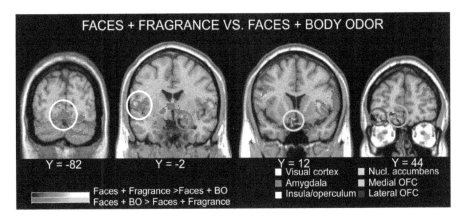

Figure 5. Group results (n=16 participants) for brain regions showing differences in brain activation when the same set of faces was presented together with the pleasant fragrance compared to the unpleasant body odor. The contrast [Faces + Fragrance > Faces + BO] is rendered in orange/yellow and the contrast [Faces + BO > Faces + Fragrance] is rendered in blue. The presence of the fragrance preferentially engaged the OFC and ventral striatum. Conversely, the unpleasant odor caused stronger activation in the amygdala, insular cortex, and visual cortex. The right side of each slice corresponds to the right side of the brain.

Conversely, a different network of brain regions responded more strongly when the faces were presented together with the unpleasant body odor. The presence of the unpleasant odor caused significantly stronger activation in the amygdala (*x/y/z* = 20/-8/-16; *z-score* = 3.03 and *x/y/z* = -18/-6/-16; *z-score* = 2.65) and anterior insular cortex (*x/y/z* = 36/12/6; *z-score* = 3.95 and *x/y/z* = -32/24/0; *z-score* = 3.01). Furthermore, we observed significantly stronger responses in the thalamus (*x/y/z* = 12/-16/4; *z-score* = 3.95 and *x/y/z* = -6/-20/4; *z-score* = 3.39) and an extensive cluster located at the junction of the rolandic operculum with the superior temporal sulcus (*x/y/z* = 60/-22/18; *z-score* = 4.06 and *x/y/z* = -62/-20/-14; *z-score* = 3.79). The only differences in frontal brain regions was found in the right medial frontal gyrus (*x/y/z* = 30/28/30; *z-score* = 2.69). Interestingly, both visual cortical areas (*x/y/z* = -2/-86/-10; *z-score* = 3.02) as well as the cerebellum (x/y/z = 12/-56/-14; z-score = 3.50 and x/y/z = -20/-60/-20; z-score = 3.97) also displayed stronger activation when the faces were accompanied by the unpleasant odor. A further analysis of the percentage BOLD signal change in the peak activated voxels in the amygdala (see Figure 7) revealed positive signal changes for all conditions.

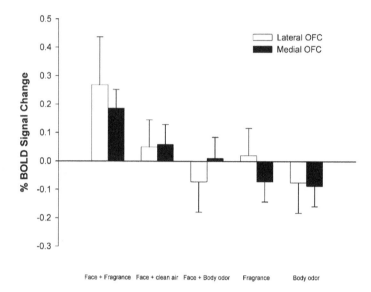

Figure 6. The average (n=16 participants) percentage BOLD signal change in the peak voxels in both medial and lateral OFC are shown for each of the five experimental conditions. Error bars depict the standard error.

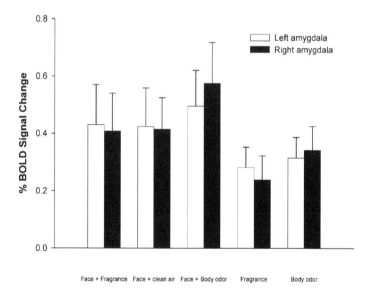

Figure 7. The average (n=16 participants) percentage BOLD signal change from baseline in the peak voxels in both the left and right amygdala are shown for each of the five experimental conditions. Error bars depict the standard error.

4. Discussion

The principal aim of the present study was to determine whether specific pleasant vs. unpleasant odors can exert a significant influence on the perception of facial attractiveness. Behavioral results confirmed that the two odors used in this study (a male fragrance and a synthetic body odor) were indeed perceived as different with respect to their pleasantness. Significantly, when briefly presented with the same set of male faces, the female participants in this study judged the faces accompanied by the pleasant fragrance as more attractive than when the faces were presented with an unpleasant synthetic body odor. This effect was related to a modulatory effect exerted by the unpleasant odor, as no significant difference in facial attractiveness *ratings* was found between the pleasant odor and a 'no odor' control condition.

In agreement with the behavioral data, the pleasant fragrance activated the medial OFC, a region that encodes the reward value of stimuli across a variety of sensory modalities including olfaction [27, 30, 39, 40]. Conversely, the unpleasant odor activated a different network or brain regions, including the amygdala which has previously been implicated in the processing of aversive stimuli [30, 41, 42].

There is currently some controversy over the role of the amygdala in the processing of odor hedonics, since the established view that this region specifically encodes aversive odors [43, 42] has been challenged by several more recent studies. For example, Anderson and colleagues [27] used the pleasant odor citral (which has a lemon smell) and the unpleasant odor valeric acid (a rancid smell) in high and low concentrations so that they could vary the valence and intensity of these stimuli. They found that amygdala activation was associated with odor intensity, but was independent of valence. Conversely, activity in the OFC was associated with odor valence, independent of intensity. In a similar study using a greater number of odors (3 pleasant and 3 unpleasant), Rolls and colleagues [40] found that ratings of odor intensity were correlated with the magnitude of the BOLD signal in medial olfactory cortical areas (including the piriform and anterior entorhinal cortex), but not in the OFC. In contrast, pleasant odors were found to activate a medial region of the OFC, whereas unpleasant odors activated the left lateral OFC, irrespective of odor intensity. Activation of this area have also been reported after monetary losses, unattractiveness in face stimuli, and the presentation of aversive odors [39, 44, 45, 46]. Since the odors used in the present study were matched with respect to their intensities, this supports the notion that stimulus aversiveness is encoded in the human amygdala. This view is also supported by the results of a recent study demonstrating that the amygdala does not encode odor valence or intensity *per se*, but rather appears to contain a general representation of the emotional value of a stimulus [47].

When the activation seen in response to more attractive faces was compared to that seen in response to relatively less attractive faces, it was found that the former engaged a reward circuit consisting of the medial OFC and nucleus accumbens, consistent with previous studies [31, 14, 15]. By contrast, relatively less attractive faces gave rise to stronger activation in the amygdala, a region implicated in the processing of the emotional expression of faces [48, 49] particularly when the expression is negative (fear, anger). The results presented here suggest that less attractive faces produce a similar neural response to that elicited by faces displaying negative emotions.

The main finding to emerge from this study was that the presence of odors with different hedonic characteristics altered the perception of male facial attractiveness in female participants. Under such conditions of bimodal stimulation, we found that when the faces were presented together with a pleasant fragrance, increased BOLD activation was predominantly observed in the OFC and ventral striatum (i.e. in the same regions that are engaged when viewing attractive faces). It appears that the positive valence of the odor interacted with the representation (itself not unpleasant), with the neuroimaging data providing a more in these regions, leading to an overall positive emotional response to the multisensory combination of stimuli (i.e., face plus odor). This observation is consistent with previous studies that have implicated these regions in the processing of facial attractiveness [31, 14, 15] and positively valenced odors [27, 40, 47]. Despite the observation that attractiveness *ratings* were no different when faces were presented together with the pleasant odor compared to faces presented in the absence of odors, significantly positive BOLD responses within the OFC were only observed in the former condition. This may suggest that even though the pleasant odor did not increase the consciously perceived and reported visual attractiveness of the faces *per se*, the medial OFC did and here we conjecture that this effect engaged more implicit affective processes that participants were unable to access consciously, but would nonetheless impact on mechanisms underpinning liking.

In contrast, when the male faces were presented with the unpleasant body odor, ratings of facial attractiveness were significantly reduced, compared to the pleasant odor and the odorless condition. The presence of the unpleasant odor caused significantly stronger activation in the insular cortex and the amygdala, both of which have previously been implicated in the representation of negative affect [50, 51, 52] and facial unattractiveness [15]. It thus appears that the aversiveness of the body odor negatively influences the emotional response to a face, leading to a decrease in its perceived attractiveness, an effect that was observed for faces of both high and low attractiveness. Several factors might explain the observation that the body odor influenced the ratings and brain activation more strongly than the fragrance. First, the hedonic difference of the body odor from hedonically neutral was greater than that of the fragrance (rating of 1.78 for body odor versus. 3.68 for fragrance with 3 being 'neutral'), so that a stronger effect might be expected on that basis alone.

In conclusion, even though the behavioral response (as measured by overt rating of facial attractiveness) in the presence of the pleasant odor, or no odor, condition did not influence facial attractiveness, results from the neuroimaging component of the study did show activations in the reward processing areas of OFC and ventral striatum. Reward region activity as evaluated using fMRI did not therefore follow the results of the behavioural task. The latter, we suggest, lacked the sensitivity required to dissociate between the fragrance and clean air (itself not unpleasant) of facial attractiveness with the neuroimaging data providing a more sensitive measure of affective state. For the unpleasant body odor, our findings support the notion that in the context of facial beauty, unpleasant odors have higher overt emotional salience than pleasant odors.

Acknowledgements

We would like to thank Unilever Research for supporting this research.

Author details

Francis McGlone[1], Robert A. Österbauer[2], Luisa M. Demattè[3] and Charles Spence[3]

1 School of Natural Sciences and Psychology, Liverpool John Moores University, UK

2 Oxford Centre for Functional Magnetic Resonance Imaging of the Brain, John Radcliffe Hospital, University of Oxford, Oxford, UK

3 Crossmodal Research Laboratory, Department of Experimental Psychology, University of Oxford, Oxford, UK

References

[1] Frieze IH, Olson JE and, Good DC, Perceived and actual discrimination in the salaries of male and female managers. *J. Appl. Soc. Psychol* 20: 46–67, 1990

[2] Marlowe CM, Schneider SL, and Nelson CE. Gender and attractiveness biases in hiring decisions are more experienced managers less biased? *J. Appl. Psychol* 81: 11–21, 1996

[3] Perrett DI, Lee KJ, Penton-Voak I, Rowland D, Yoshikawa S, Burt DM, Henzi SP, Castles DL, and Akamatsu S. Effects of sexual dimorphism on facial attractiveness. *Nature* 394: 884-887, 1998.

[4] Grammer K, and Thornhill R. Human (Homo sapiens) facial attractiveness and sexual selection: the role of symmetry and averageness. *J Comp Psychol* 108: 233-242, 1994.

[5] Hoss RA, Ramsey JL, Griffin AM, and Langlois JH. The role of facial attractiveness and facial masculinity/femininity in sex classification of faces. *Perception* 34: 1459-1474, 2005.

[6] Perrett D, May K, and Yoshikawa S. Facial shape and judgments of female attractiveness. *Nature 368*: 239–242, 1994.

[7] Adolphs R, Tranel D, Damasio H, and Damasio A. Impaired recognition of emotion in facial expressions following bilateral damage to the human amygdala. *Nature* 372: 669-672, 1994.

[8]   Blair RJ, Morris JS, Frith CD, Perrett DI, and Dolan RJ. Dissociable neural responses to facial expressions of sadness and anger. *Brain* 122: 883-893, 1999.

[9]   Haxby JV, Hoffman EA, and Gobbini MI. Human neural systems for face recognition and social communication. *Biol Psychiatry* 51: 59-67, 2002.

[10] Morris JS, Frith CD, Perrett DI, Rowland D, Young AW, Calder AJ, and Dolan RJ. A differential neural response in the human amygdala to fearful and happy facial expressions. *Nature* 383: 812-815, 1996.

[11] Posamentier MT, and Abdi H. Processing faces and facial expressions. *Neuropsychol Rev* 13: 113-143, 2003.

[12] Nakamura K, Kawashima R, Nagumo S, Ito K, Sugiura M, Kato T, Nakamura A, Hatano K, Kubota K, Fukuda H, and Kojima S. Neuroanatomical correlates of the assessment of facial attractiveness. *Neuroreport* 9: 753-757, 1998

[13] Aharon I, Etcoff N, Ariely D, Chabris CF, O'Connor E, and Breiter HC. Beautiful faces have variable reward value: fMRI and behavioral evidence. *Neuron* 32: 537-551, 2001.

[14] Kampe KK, Frith CD, Dolan RJ, and Frith U. Reward value of attractiveness and gaze. *Nature* 413: 589, 2001.

[15] O'Doherty J, Winston J, Critchley H, Perrett D, Burt DM, and Dolan RJ. Beauty in a smile: the role of medial orbitofrontal cortex in facial attractiveness. *Neuropsychologia* 41: 147-155, 2003.

[16] Casey SJ, Woods AT, and Newell FN. Is beauty in the eyes and ear of the beholder? In: *7th Annual Meeting of the International Multisensory Research Forum*. Dublin, Ireland: 200

[17] Zuckerman M, Miyake K, and Hodgins HS. Cross-channel effects of vocal and physical attractiveness and their implications for interpersonal perception. *J Pers Soc Psychol* 60: 545-554, 1991.

[18] Rikowski A, and Grammer K. Human body odour, symmetry and attractiveness. *Proc Biol Sci* 266: 869-874, 1999.

[19] Kovács G, Gulyas B, Savic I, Perrett DI, Cornwell RE, Little AC, Jones BC, Burt DM, Gal V, and Vidnyanszky Z. Smelling human sex hormone-like compounds affects face gender judgment of men. *Neuroreport* 15: 1275-1277, 2004.

[20] Dematte ML, Osterbauer R, and Spence C. Olfactory cues modulate facial attractiveness. *Chem Senses* 32: 603-610, 2007.

[21] Gottfried JA, O'Doherty J, and Dolan RJ. Appetitive and aversive olfactory learning in humans studied using event-related functional magnetic resonance imaging. *J Neurosci* 22: 10829-10837, 2002.

[22] König R. Kulturanthropologische Betrachtungen zum Problem der Parfmierung [A cultural anthropological consideration of the problem of perfume]. *J Cosmet Sci* 23: 823-829, 1972.

[23] Gottfried JA, and Dolan RJ. The nose smells what the eye sees: crossmodal visual facilitation of human olfactory perception. *Neuron* 39: 375-386, 2003

[24] Morrot G, Brochet F, and Dubourdieu D. The color of odors. *Brain Lang* 79: 309-320, 2001.

[25] Österbauer RA, Matthews PM, Jenkinson M, Beckmann CF, Hansen PC, and Calvert GA. Color of scents: chromatic stimuli modulate odor responses in the human brain. *J Neurophysiol* 93: 3434-3441, 2005.

[26] Zellner DA, Bartoli AM, and Eckard R. Influence of color on odor identification and liking ratings. *Am J Psychol* 104: 547-561, 1991.

[27] Anderson AK, Christoff K, Stappen I, Panitz D, Ghahremani DG, Glover G, Gabrieli JD, and Sobel N. Dissociated neural representations of intensity and valence in human olfaction. *Nat Neurosci* 6: 196-202, 2003.

[28] de Araujo IE, Rolls ET, Kringelbach ML, McGlone F, and Phillips N. Taste-olfactory convergence, and the representation of the pleasantness of flavour, in the human brain. *Eur J Neurosci* 18: 2059-2068, 2003.

[29] de Araujo IE, Rolls ET, Velazco MI, Margot C, and Cayeux I. Cognitive modulation of olfactory processing. *Neuron* 46: 671-679, 2005.

[30] Gottfried JA, O'Doherty J, and Dolan RJ. Encoding predictive reward value in human amygdala and orbitofrontal cortex. *Science* 301: 1104-1107, 2003.

[31] Ishai A. Sex, beauty and the orbitofrontal cortex. *Int J Psychophysiol* 63: 181-185, 2006

[32] Schneider W, Eschman A, and Zuccolotto A. *E-Prime reference guide. Pittsburgh, PA: Psychology Software Tools Inc.* 2002.

[33] Jenkinson M, Bannister P, Brady M, and Smith S. Improved optimization for the robust and accurate linear registration and motion correction of brain images. *Neuroimage* 17: 825-841, 2002.

[34] Woolrich MW, Ripley BD, Brady M, and Smith SM. Temporal autocorrelation in univariate linear modeling of FMRI data. *Neuroimage* 14: 1370-1386, 2001.

[35] Beckmann CF, Jenkinson M, and Smith SM. General multilevel linear modeling for group analysis in FMRI. *Neuroimage* 20: 1052-1063, 2003.

[36] Forman SD, Cohen JD, Fitzgerald M, Eddy WF, Mintun MA, and Noll DC. Improved assessment of significant activation in functional magnetic resonance imaging (fMRI): use of a cluster-size threshold. *Magn Reson Med* 33: 636-647, 1995.

[37] Friston KJ, Worsley KJ, Frakowiak RSJ, Mazziotta JC, and Evans AC. Assessing the significance of focal activations using their spatial extent. *Hum Brain Mapp* 1: 214-220, 1994.

[38] Worsley KJ, Evans AC, Marrett S, and Neelin P. A three-dimensional statistical analysis for CBF activation studies in human brain. *J Cereb Blood Flow Metab* 12: 900-918, 1992.

[39] O'Doherty J, Rolls ET, Francis S, Bowtell R, and McGlone F. Representation of pleasant and aversive taste in the human brain. *J Neurophysiol* 85: 1315-1321, 2001.

[40] Rolls ET, Kringelbach ML, and de Araujo IE. Different representations of pleasant and unpleasant odours in the human brain. *Eur J Neurosci* 18: 695-703, 2003.

[41] Zald DH, Lee JT, Fluegel KW, and Pardo JV. Aversive gustatory stimulation activates limbic circuits in humans. *Brain* 121: 1143-1154, 1998.

[42] Zald DH, and Pardo JV. Emotion, olfaction, and the human amygdala: amygdala activation during aversive olfactory stimulation. *Proc Natl Acad Sci USA* 94: 4119-4124, 1997.

[43] Royet JP, Hudry J, Zald DH, Godinot D, Gregoire MC, Lavenne F, Costes N, and Holley A. Functional neuroanatomy of different olfactory judgments. *Neuroimage* 13: 506-519, 2001.

[44] Ursu, S. and Carter, C. S. Outcome representations, counterfactual comparisons and the human orbitofrontal cortex: implications for neuroimaging studies of decision-making. *Cogn Brain Res*, 23(1), 51-60, 2005

[45] Liu X, Powell DK, Wang H, Gold BT, Corbly CR, and Joseph JE. Functional dissociation in frontal and striatal areas for processing of positive and negative reward information. *J Neurosci* 27:4587– 4597, 2007

[46] Elloit R, Agnew Z, and Deakin B. Hedonic and Informational Functions of the Human Orbitofrontal Cortex. *Cerebral Cortex* 20(1): 198-204, 2010

[47] Winston JS, Gottfried JA, Kilner JM, and Dolan RJ. Integrated neural representations of odor intensity and affective valence in human amygdala. *J Neurosci* 25: 8903-8907, 2005.

[48] Dolan RJ, Morris JS, and de Gelder B. Crossmodal binding of fear in voice and face. *Proc Natl Acad Sci USA* 98: 10006-10010, 2001.

[49] Kesler-West ML, Andersen AH, Smith CD, Avison MJ, Davis CE, Kryscio RJ, and Blonder LX. Neural substrates of facial emotion processing using fMRI. *Brain Res Cogn Brain Res* 11: 213-226, 2001.

[50] Nitschke JB, Sarinopoulos I, Mackiewicz KL, Schaefer HS, and Davidson RJ. Functional neuroanatomy of aversion and its anticipation. *Neuroimage* 29: 106-116, 2006.

[51] Sato W, Yoshikawa S, Kochiyama T, and Matsumura M. The amygdala processes the emotional significance of facial expressions: an fMRI investigation using the interaction between expression and face direction. *Neuroimage* 22: 1006-1013, 2004.

[52] Wicker B, Keysers C, Plailly J, Royet JP, Gallese V, and Rizzolatti G. Both of us disgusted in my insula: the common neural basis of seeing and feeling disgust. *Neuron* 40: 655-664, 2003.

Chapter 2

Surgical Resection of Tumors Infiltrating Left Insula and Perisylvian Opercula — Utility of Anatomic Landmarks Implemented by Intraoperative Functional Brain Mapping

Francesco Signorelli, Domenico Chirchiglia,
Rodolfo Maduri, Giuseppe Barbagallo and
Jacques Guyotat

Additional information is available at the end of the chapter

1. Introduction

Tumors involving the insular lobe and perisylvian opercula of the dominant hemisphere are frequently managed conservatively regardless of their nature and clinical evolution, even if impending infiltration of nearby eloquent areas endangers their function. Our and other authors' experience (Duffau 2009, Duffau et al, 2000; 2001; 2006; 2009; Lang et al, 2001; Kim et al, 2002; Moshel et al, 2008; Saito et al, 2010; Sanai et al, 2010; Signorelli et al, 2010; 2011; Simon et al, 2009; Skrap et al, 2012; Yasargil et al, 1992; Wu et al, 2011; Zentner et al, 1996) demonstrate that wide surgical resection of these lesions are nonetheless feasible since tumor burden often displaces eloquent sites at the tumor boundaries (Duffau 2000; Duffau et al, 2000; 2001; 2006; 2009; Signorelli et al, 2010; 2011) and compensatory areas take over the lost function of infiltrated nervous tissue. However, accurate anatomic and functional knowledge of the sylvian fissure and structures located nearby is essential to perform any surgical act in this area, in order to decrease the risks of postoperative permanent deficits (Duffau 2009; Duffau et al, 2009; Moshel et al, 2009; Signorelli et al, 2010; 2011). Here we report our recent experience with tumors infiltrating left insula and perisylvian opercula and point out technical details helpful in guiding surgery through this region, with the purpose of locating and respecting neural and vascular structures and eloquent sites.

Surgical Resection of Tumors Infiltrating Left Insula and Perisylvian Opercula — Utility of Anatomic
Landmarks Implemented by Intraoperative Functional Brain Mapping

21

2. Patients and methods

Our series includes 5 patients harboring a high grade and 10 patients harboring a low grade tumor involving left insula and perisylvian opercula, operated on between 2007 and 2011 at two institutions: the Neurosurgical Department at the Hôpital Neurologique et Neurochirurgical "Pierre Wertheimer" in Lyon, France, and the Neurosurgical Department of the University Hospital of Catanzaro, Italy. They were 8 males and 7 females (mean age 50.1 years) who presented with phasic troubles in 8 cases and seizures in all cases. Preoperative antiepileptic treatment was effective in all patients but one, although 3 other patients presented with more than 1 seizure/month. Aphasia was completely regressive in four patients, all LGG, and partially regressive in one HGG patient after administration of antiedema therapy and seizure control, while in 3 other HGG cases it was progressive at a thorough preoperative neuropsychologic evaluation which comprised Montreal-Toulouse and Boston tests (Dordain et al, 1983) repeated at 1-month. They were nonetheless judged to be good candidates for, and keen and motivated to undergo intraoperative language mapping.

Motor deficit was a presenting symptom in two patients. Moreover, in all HGG patients there were symptoms of intracranial hypertension (ICHT). ICHT had an acute onset in one patient which presented to our department with an intratumoral hemorrhage. This last patient displayed a right sensorimotor deficit and a right homonymous hemianopia. Surgical indication was established in lesions with a MRI appearance of LGG in two cases because of clinical and/or radiological tumor progression and in the other eight cases at the time of diagnosis.. All patients were right handed according to the Edimburgh Handedness Inventory (Oldfield, 1971). Gadolinium-enhanced T1-, T2- and FLAIR-weighted images revealed in all cases the infiltration of left insula. The tumor involved also fronto-parietal and temporal opercula in 9 cases, while frontal and temporal opercula or just parietal or temporal operculum were infiltrated respectively in three, two and one case. Moreover, the tumor infiltrated other paralimbic structures (i.e. fronto-orbital and/or temporo-polar areas) in four cases and limbic structures in two cases. In order to elucidate the relationships of the tumor with the vascular tree of left middle cerebral artery (MCA), in particular with lenticulostriate arteries, left carotid angiography was obtained for two patient. The other 13 patients underwent angio-CT scan and/or MRI angiography. The most lateral lenticulostiate branch was shown in 3 out of 15 cases originating from the post-bifurcation tract of M1, no more than 6 mm distal from the major bifurcation, while in the other cases it originated before or at the level of the MCA bifurcation but never from M2, in accordance with other author's experience (Moshel et al, 2008). Particular attention was also paid to the venograms, to determine the course of the superficial sylvian veins, which can hinder a wide dissection of the sylvian fissure, although generally sylvian fissure was approached subpially.

2.1. Surgical procedure

All patients underwent awake craniotomy using electrical stimulation mapping (ESM) of sensorimotor and language pathways, whose technique was described in detail elsewhere (Signorelli et al, 2010; 2011). Briefly, we applied a bipolar cortico-subcortical stimulation by an electrode with tips 5 mm apart, which delivered biphasic square-wave pulses (1 ms per phase) with a frequency of 60 pulses per second. Cortical stimulation was started at 1 mA and the optimal current level for stimulation was set equal to that provoking segmental movements on the contralateral upper limb or face. The effective current intensity varied from 1 mA to 6 mA. Language tasks included counting, verbal and auditory naming (auditory task was used when testing anterior temporal lobe sites). Moreover, reading tasks were added when testing parietal or posterior temporal opercula. Neuronavigation was used for all patients for defining tumor boundaries and anatomic relationships with neural and vascular structures. Craniotomy was planned to include the whole perisylvian area from pars orbitalis of the third frontal gyrus to the postcentral sulcus, in order to expose the anterior (vallecula) and middle part (insular fossa) of the sylvian fissure, exposing also the superior temporal gyrus (T1). After performing ESM aimed at locating cortical language and sensorimotor areas, the superficial part of the lesion, which constantly infiltrated one or more of frontal, parietal and temporal opercula, was removed as to gain easy access to the depth of sylvian fissure, which was opened up to the postcentral sulcus with no need of retractors. In all our cases the tumor displaced M2 branches centrifugally, indicating to the surgeon the site on the insular surface where to start tumor debulking, after accomplishment of ESM in search of possible language areas. The removal of insular gyri, when not harboring language areas, was conducted medially up to the putamen, generally visible under the microscope as a gray, compact tissue with white strips located at the center of insula (Yasargyl et al, 1992), which we never found infiltrated in case of low grade tumors. However, while pushing medially tumor removal, we alternated surgical resection to subcortical stimulation starting at a distance of 2 cm laterally to the posterior limb of the internal capsule, as seen on neuronavigation, in order to identify and preserve subcortical motor pathways (Duffau 2009; Signorelli et al, 2010; 2011; Simon et al, 2009;). Subcortical stimulation is especially useful when pushing tumor resection above superior insular sulcus, where pyramidal fibers coursing through corona radiata are more superficial and anatomic landmarks to them lack. High attention was paid when pushing resection below the lenticular nucleus, at the level of the inferior limiting sulcus, where sublenticular fibers of the posterior limb of the internal capsule contain, in a forward-backward direction, the auditory and the optic radiations (Signorelli et al, 2010). At the level of the anterior part of the external capsule subcortical stimulation allowed the identification of the inferior occipito-frontal fasciculus inducing semantic paraphasias (Duffau 2009), which delimited the deep boundaries of tumor resection anteriorly. The temporal part of the same fasciculus marked the boundaries of the resection at the level of the temporal stem, preventing to open the temporal horn of the ventricle (Duffau 2009; Duffau et a, 2009). Of utmost importance is the recognition of the vascular anatomy. Short branches from MCA to the infiltrated insula can be interrupted because they supply the tumor, paying attention not to avulse them from the main vessel at the origin, which can lead to a lesion of the parent vessel wall. However, long perforators, supplying corona radiata, have to be respected to avoid ischemic injury to functional white matter (Duffau 2009; Lang et al, 2001; Moshel et al, 2008; Signorelli et al, 2010; 2011). During removal of limen insulae high attention has to be paid to lenticulostriate arteries, which originates mostly from the medial or superior aspect of MCA 6 mm or less around bifurcation and sometimes from

Surgical Resection of Tumors Infiltrating Left Insula and Perisylvian Opercula — Utility of Anatomic
Landmarks Implemented by Intraoperative Functional Brain Mapping

23

early M1 branches (Signorelli et al 2010). Lesion or even manipulation of them can lead to ischemic damage of the internal capsule.

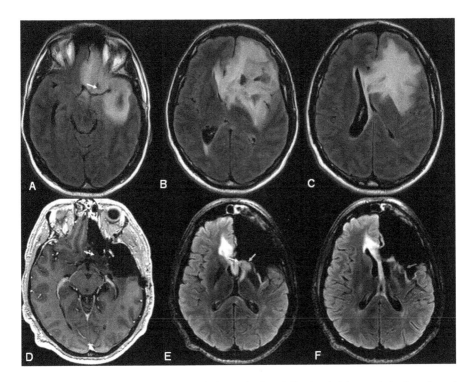

Figure 1. A, B,C: Preoperative FLAIR MR images of a low grade glioma infiltrating the left operculo-insular region and the fronto-orbital, including the perforated substance (white arrow), temporopolar and hyppocampal regions, type 5 B of Yasargil classification (Yasargil et al, 1992). **D**: Postoperative T1 gadolinium-weighted and **E,F**: Postoperative FLAIR MR images, showing the subtotal removal of the lesion. The boundaries of the resection are set based on anatomical (perforated substance, white arrow) as well as neurofunctional (subcallosal fasciculus, yellow arrow; inferior occipitofrontal fasciculus, green arrow; arcuate fasciculus, blue arrow) criteria.

3. Results

3.1. Electrophysiological results

ESM of the insular cortex surface resulted in speech arrest in 6 patients In 9 patients insula was free of language sites, as it was in all cases the cortex of opercular clefts and of superior and inferior insular clefts. For what concerns the location of eloquent sites at the level of the convexity, ESM located essential language sites on immediately perisylvian tumoral tissue in just one patient, while in the rest of cases functional areas were displaced at the periphery of grossly infiltrated nervous tissue. The insular cortical areas whose stimulation evoked abdominal sensations such as nausea, borborygmi, belching (2 patients), chewing and tongue movements without speech arrest (4 patients) were not considered eloquent sites and removed because infiltrated by tumor. In one case ESM caused intraoperative partial tonic-clonic seizures, rapidly stopped pouring cold serum on the cortex. A gross total removal was achieved in all 6 patients that did not display infiltration of perisylvian or insular functional cortex and subcortical motor or language pathways. Stimulation of uncinate fasciculus during removal of an infiltrated limen insulae was done in 8 patients and was always uneventful. In all patients stimulation of the infiltrated white matter at the anterolateral border of the frontal horn of the left lateral ventricle (i.e. the subcallosal fasciculus) triggered limited spontaneous speech and/or perseverations with preservation of normal articulation and at the level of the anterior part of the external capsule as well as at the level of the temporal stem induced semantic paraphasias, which delimited the deep boundaries of tumor resection. Moreover, ESM was used to identify motor pathways inside corona radiata above the insular superior limiting sulcus, which represented the posterosuperior limit of tumor resection.

3.2. Clinical results

Ten patients had an immediate postoperative phasic aggravation, which lasted 1 to 2 months. At an overall mean follow up of 33 months (14-56 months) 10 patients are alive and keep a good quality of life, as assessed by the EORTC QLQ-C30 (Aaronson et al, 1993). One of them presents a tumor relapse, which causes an impairment of language performances, but she is still autonomous. Seven patients keep the same functional status they had before intervention, while two patients display an improvement of their neuropsychological performance after surgery. Three of the five patients diagnosed with a HGG died after a mean survival period of 16.7 months. Two of them had a mean HQSP (high quality survival period) of 18 months, while the last patient had a postoperative nucleo-capsular infarct, due to lenticulostriate arteries damage, engendering a definitive motor and phasic aggravation. Two other HGG patients, with a follow-up of 23 and 6 months respectively, are autonomous and have a good quality of life. For what concerns seizures outcome, 9 patients were ameliorated and 6 had no variation as regards to their preoperative status. On the postoperative MRI resection was in 6 cases grossly total, in 6 cases subtotal and in three cases partial owing to tumoral infiltration of functional tissue.

4. Discussion

Several well designed controlled studies indicate that the degree of surgical resection of brain gliomas, including those in highly eloquent areas, affects survival and quality of life of patients (Duffau 2009; Ius et al, 2012; Sanai et al, 2010) and there are some good reasons to treat aggressively such tumors: cytoreduction is effective in reducing the mass effect of the lesion and it can be assumed that it reduces also the contingent of neoplastic cells that can reproduce and give origin to tumor recurrence and invasion of eloquent areas or take anaplastic trans-formation (Duffau 2009; Ius et al, 2012; Sanai et al, 2010). Moreover, there are evidences that aggressive removal of insular tumors can improve seizures control, which are their most frequent clinical manifestation (Taillandier et al, 2009). Authors pleading for an aggressive treatment of such tumors mostly think that it should be realized early after diagnosis to prevent clinical impairment and improve survival and recurrence free period of patients (Duffau 2009; Sanai et al, 2010).

Since the first report by Yasargil et al, other papers in the literature dealt with the surgical treatment of tumors infiltrating insular lobe (Duffau 2009, Duffau et al, 2000; 2001; 2006; 2009; Lang et al, 2001; Kim et al, 2002; Moshel et al, 2008; Saito et al, 2010; Sanai et al, 2010; Signorelli et al, 2010; 2011; Simon et al, 2009; Skrap et al, 2012; Yasargil et al, 1992; Wu et al, 2011; Zentner et al, 1996) and encompassed lesions with a variety of anatomical extensions. As a matter of fact, these series reported on purely insular tumors (type 3A of the Yasargyl's classification) as well as insulo-opercular (type 3B) and limbic-paralimbic lesions (type 5) involving both the dominant and the non-dominant hemisphere. Some authors reporting surgical removal of dominant-sided insular tumors did not find useful or did not employ awake surgery for language mapping (Hentschel et al, 2005; Lang et al, 2001; Simon et al, 2009; Yasargyl et al, 1992; Zentner et al, 1996), others demonstrated the utility of ESM mapping guided tumor resection, although seldom insula was found to harbor essential language sites (Duffau 2009; Duffau et al, 2001; 2009). In Duffau's series there were no permanent postoperative phasic deficits although he reported 10 cases of transient articulatory disorders (Duffau et al, 2000). In Hentschel and Lang's series there were 6 cases of transient speech troubles among patients with 3B tumors and in Zentner's series two of the 11 patients had a permanent postoperative aphasia (Hentschel et al, 2005; Zentner et al, 1996).

Our series, albeit small, is anatomically homogeneous in that focuses on tumors infiltrating the insular lobe of the dominant hemisphere and extended to the opercular region and, in six cases, also to adjacent deep perisylvian structures. Moreover, all patients were operated on while testing language function. The retrospective analysis restricted to these patients shows two basic findings: 6 out of 15 such patients, all harboring a LGG infiltrating the frontoparietal and temporal opercula, had speech arrest while stimulating insular cortex and these same patients did not have language sites on the opercular part invaded by the tumor. Conversely, the 9 patients for whom ESM of insular cortex did not trigger language troubles all harboured speech function on perisylvian opercula. They either had preoperative language troubles (4 cases), which did not hinder intraoperative language mapping, or a limited opercular infil-tration, and no phasic deficits (5 cases).Thus, it can be speculated that for the 6 LGG patients displaying language sites on insula, this region compensated the opercular infiltration due to a plasticity phenomenon, which can be considered at least in part responsible for the preop-erative regression of the phasic deficits. For the remaining patients the functional reorganiza-tion might not have occurred because of a limited opercular infiltration (1 patient) or because of a too extensive and rapid inactivation of perisylvian language sites by a high grade tumor. The compensatory role of left insula in case of infiltration of perisylvian language areas has already been pointed out as a function that must be preserved (Duffau et al, 2000). However, the compensatory potential of left insula seems to be highly variable on individual basis. There are mechanisms of cerebral plasticity taking place before the treatment of the lesion and both in an acute stage and at distance from surgical intervention. This could be explained by the fact that sensorimotor and language functions seem to be organised within multiple parallel networks. Beyond the recruitment of areas adjacent to the surgical cavity, the long term reshaping could be related to progressive involvement of regions within the hemisphere omolateral to the lesion as well as of the contralateral hemisphere (Duffau, 2006).. In these cases functional reshaping involves association areas belonging to the same functional network of the lesioned area as it is the case for dominant insula and perisilvyan language sites. However, mechanisms of compensation are limited. One of such limits is that reorganisation seems to be more effective in secondary than in primary areas, as for SMA (Duffau, 2006). Moreover, if a damaged area is compensated by another region, a lesion of this newly recruited region will induce a permanent deficit, as it could be the case for dominant insulo-opercular gliomas. Thus, surgical resection should avoid infringement of insula if there are arguments indicating that it took over, at least partially, the lost function of perisylvian opercula. Taking into account these data may guide treatment of cerebral tumors in the dominant deep perisylvian area, broadening the surgical indication and the extent of tumor removal while lessening the rate of postoperative permanent deficits, and be useful for defining prognosis and rehabilitation programs.

Abbreviations

ESM: electrical stimulation mapping; HGG: high grade gliomas; ICHT: intracranial hypertension; LGG: low grade gliomas; MCA: middle cerebral artery; MRI: magnetic resonance imaging; T1: superior temporal gyrus.

Author details

Francesco Signorelli[1,2], Domenico Chirchiglia[3], Rodolfo Maduri[1], Giuseppe Barbagallo[4] and Jacques Guyotat[1]

1 "Magna Græcia" University, Department of Experimental and Clinical Medicine "G. Salvatore", Chair of Neurosurgery, Catanzaro, Italy

2 Hospices Civils de Lyon, Hôpital Neurologique et Neurochirurgical, Department of Neurosurgery, Lyon, France

3 "Magna Græcia" University, Department of Medical and Surgical Sciences, Chair of Neurosurgery, Catanzaro, Italy

4 University of Catania, Chair of Neurosurgery, Catania, Italy

References

[1] Aaronson, N. K, Ahmedzai, S, Bergman, B, Bullinger, M, Cull, A, Duez, N. J, Filiberti, A, Flechtner, H, Fleishman, S. B, De Haes, J. C, et al. The European Organization for Research and Treatment of Cancer QLQ-C30: AQuality-of-Life Instrument for Use in International Clinical Trials in Oncology. Journal of the National Cancer Institute. (1993). , 85, 365-376.

[2] Dordain, M, Nespoulos, J. L, & Bourdeau, M. Lecours AR Verbal abilities of normal adults submitting to an aphasia linguistic protocol. Acta Neurol Belg. (1983).

[3] Duffau H, Capelle L, Lopes M, Faillot T, Sichez JP, Fohanno D. The insular lobe: physiopathological and surgical considerations. *Neurosurgery.* 2000;47:801-10.

[4] Duffau H, Bauchet L, Lehéricy S, Capelle L. Functional compensation of the left dominant insula for language. *Neuroreport.* 2001. 20;12:2159-63.

[5] Duffau H, Taillandier L, Gatignol P, Capelle L. The insular lobe and brain plasticity: Lessons from tumor surgery. *Clin Neurol Neurosurg.* 2006;108:543-8.

[6] Duffau, H. Lessons from brain mapping in surgery for low grade gliomas: study of cerebral connectivity and plasticity. In Medical Imaging and Augmented Reality. (2006). Online 978-3-54037-221-9Springer Berlin Heidelberg.

[7] Duffau H, Moritz-Gasser S, Gatignol P. Functional outcome after language mapping for insular World Health Organization Grade II gliomas in the dominant hemisphere: experience with 24 patients. *Neurosurg Focus.* 2009;27(2):E.

[8] Duffau, H. A personal consecutive series of surgically treated 51 cases of insular WHO Grade II glioma: advances and limitations. J Neurosurg. (2009). , 110, 696-708.

[9] Hentschel SJ, Lang FF. Surgical resection of intrinsic insular tumors. *Neurosurgery.* 2005;57:176-83.

[10] Ius T, Isola M, Budai R, Pauletto G, Tomasino B, Fadiga L, Skrap M. Low-grade glioma surgery in eloquent areas: volumetric analysis of extent of resection and its impact on overall survival. A single-institution experience in 190 patients: clinical article. *J Neurosurg.* 2012;117:1039-52.

[11] Kim YH, Kim CY.Current surgical management of insular gliomas. *Neurosurg Clin N Am.* 2012;23:199-206,

[12] Lang FF, Olansen NE, DeMonte F, Gokaslan ZL, Holland EC, Kalhorn C, Sawaya R. Surgical resection of intrinsic insular tumors: complication avoidance. *J Neurosurg.* 2001 Oct;95(4):638-50.

[13] Moshel YA, Marcus JD, Parker EC, Kelly PJ. Resection of insular gliomas: the importance of lenticulostriate artery position. *J Neurosurg.* 2008 Nov;109(5):825-34.

[14] Oldfield, R. C. The assessment and analysis of handedness: The Edinburgh invento-
      ry. Neuropsychologia. (1971). , 9, 97-113.

[15] Saito R, Kumabe T, Kanamori M, Sonoda Y, Tominaga T. Insulo-opercular gliomas:
      four different natural progression patterns and implications for surgical indications.
      Neurol Med Chir (Tokyo). 2010;50:286-90

[16] Sanai N, Polley MY, Berger MS. Insular glioma resection: assessment of patient mor-
      bidity, survival, and tumor progression. *J Neurosurg*. 2010;112:1-9.

[17] Signorelli, F.; Guyotat, J; Elisevich, K. & Barbagallo, GM. Review of current microsur-
      gical management of insular gliomas. *Acta Neurochirurgica*. 2010;152:19-26.

[18] Signorelli, F. Barbagallo, GM; Maduri R, Schonauer C, Guyotat, J, & Elisevich, K. In-
      sular tumors. In Management of CNS Tumors, (2011). 978-9-53307-646-1Ed. Miklos
      Garami, InTech- Open Access Publisher- Rijeka, Croatia.

[19] Simon M, Neuloh G, von Lehe M, Meyer B, Schramm J. Insular gliomas: the case for
      surgical management. *J Neurosurg*. 2009;110:685-95.

[20] Skrap M, Mondani M, Tomasino B, Weis L, Budai R, Pauletto G, Eleopra R, Fadiga L,
      Ius T.Surgery of insular nonenhancing gliomas: volumetric analysis of tumoral resec-
      tion, clinical outcome, and survival in a consecutive series of 66 cases. *Neurosurgery*.
      2012;70:1081-93

[21] Taillandier L, Duffau H. Epilepsy and insular Grade II gliomas: an interdisciplinary
      point of view from a retrospective monocentric series of 46 cases. *Neurosurg Focus*.
      2009 Aug;27(2):E8.

[22] Yasargil, M. G, Von Ammon, K, Cavazos, E, Doczi, T, Reeves, J. D, & Roth, P. Tu-
      mors of the limbic and paralimbic systems. Acta Neurochirurgica. (1992). , 147-149.

[23] Wu AS, Witgert ME, Lang FF, Xiao L, Bekele BN, Meyers CA, Ferson D, Wefel JS.
      Neurocognitive function before and after surgery for insular gliomas. *J Neurosurg*.
      2011;115:1115-25.

[24] Zentner, J, Meyer, B, Stangl, A, & Schramm, J. Intrinsic tumors of the insula: a pro-
      spective surgical study of 30 patients. Journal of Neurosurg. (1996). , 85, 263-271.

Chapter 3

Causal Relationships and Network Parameters in Effective Brain Connectivity

Guiomar Niso, Ernesto Pereda, Fernando Maestú,
María Gudín, Sira Carrasco and Francisco del-Pozo

Additional information is available at the end of the chapter

1. Introduction

The human brain comprises approximately 10^{11} neurons, each of which makes about 10^3 synaptic connections. This huge number of connections between individual processing elements provides the fundamental scaffold for neuronal ensembles to become transiently synchronized or functionally connected [1]. A similar complex network configuration and dynamics can also be found at the macroscopic scales of systems neuroscience and brain imaging [2]. The emergence of dynamically coupled cell assemblies represents the neurophysiological substrate for cognitive function such as perception, learning, thinking [3]. Understanding the complex network organization of the brain on the basis of neuroimaging data represents one of the most impervious challenges for systems neuroscience.

Several measures to evaluate at various scales (single cells, cortical columns, or brain areas) how the different parts of the brain communicate have been recently proposed. We can classify them, according to their symmetry, into two groups: symmetric and asymmetric measures. Symmetric measures, such as correlation, coherence, phase synchronization indexes (PLV, PLI), evaluate *functional connectivity,* i.e. statistically significant relationships between signals recorded from spatially remote neurophysiological events. On the other hand, the asymmetric ones are able to detect *effective connectivity* i.e. information flow (the influence one neuronal system exerts over another) [4], and therefore they reveal the direction of the interaction. Granger Causality (GC) belongs to this latter group.

2. Granger causality

2.1. Classical approach

A notion of causality, which is relevant for the experimental study of information transfer in neural systems, is commonly attributed to Wiener. He stated that, for two simultaneously measured signals, if one can predict the first signal better by incorporating the past information from the second signal than by using only information from the first one, then the second signal can be called *causal* to the first one [5]. However, it was the Nobel Prize laureate Clive Granger who gave a mathematical formulation of this concept [6]. He argued that, if X is influencing Y, then adding past values of the first variable (X) to the regression of the second one (Y) should improve the prediction of the latter.

To quantify such influence, the most straightforward approach consists in comparing the prediction of future values of one of the variables (say, X), by using two different models. The first one is a model where these values are forecast exclusively from the past history of this variable (e.g., a purely autoregressive (AR) model of a given order). The second one incorporates instead the past history of Y as well. Then, GC is defined by comparing the forecast errors of both models (see section 4.2), and Y is said to Granger-cause X if the error of the second model is significantly lower than that of the first one.

GC has the advantage of quantifying the information flow in the data, which is important to study the direction of the relationships between different parts of the brain. GC was first introduced in the field of economics 40 years ago. However, applications to neuroscience are rather more recent, see [7] for a review on applications to neurophysiology. One of the first studies using this concept investigated the existence of directional or causal interactions by analyzing local field potentials (LFPs) from the macaque inferotemporal cortex [8]. This method was also applied to the LFP data recorded from two separate areas (primary and higher visual areas) of the cat visual cortex, to investigate the role of bottom-up and top-down interactions in a go/no-go task [9] or in a stimulus expectancy task [10]. A frequency specific Granger causality measure was utilized in LFP recordings from somatosensory and motor cortices of macaque monkeys as they performed a motor maintenance in a visual discrimination task [11]. In human, a time-variant Granger causality measure was applied to EEG signals from the standard color-word conflict Stroop task [12]. A wide study CG's advantages for neuroscience was done in [13].

3. Magnetoencephalography (MEG)

3.1. Consent

Ethical approval was granted by the local Ethics Committee. All data were analyzed anonymously. Subjects who underwent MEG recordings for research purposes had given written informed consent before participating.

Once subjects arrived at the laboratory, they got familiar with the MEG chamber in which the recording took place and were instructed about the experimental procedure. All the recordings took place during morning hours.

3.2. MEG system

MEG recordings were obtained using a 306-channel wholehead Elekta Neuromag® MEG system (Elekta Oy, Helsinki, Finland). The system has 102 magnetometers and 204 planar gradiometers in a helmet-shaped array covering the entire scalp. Subjects were seated inside a magnetically shielded room during MEG recordings (Vacuumschmelze GmbH, Hanau, Germany).

Eye movements were monitored by simultaneously recording an electrooculogram (EOG), with three Ag/Cl electrodes, two above and below the right eye and one at the right earlobe used as ground reference.

3.3. Artifact control

Participants were seated with their head in the MEG sensor helmet, which covers the entire head except the face. Four head position indicator coils (HPI) were placed on the scalp, appropriately spaced in the region covered by the MEG helmet. The locations of the nasion, two pre-auricular points, and the four HPI coils were digitized prior to each MEG study using a 3D-digitizer (FASTRACK; Polhemus, Colchester, VT) to define the subject-specific cartesian head coordinate system. 100-200 additional anatomical points were digitized on the head surface to provide a more accurate shape of the subject's head. Once a subject was comfortably positioned in the MEG machine, short electrical signals were sent to the HPI coils to localize them with respect to the MEG sensor array. The data from the HPI coils were used to correct head movement during the session.

3.4. Subjects

The data used in this study were acquired from 8 patients suffering from frontal focal epilepsy (FE), 8 patients suffering from generalized epilepsy (GE) and 8 healthy subjects (HS). Their ages range between (FE: 35.1 ± 14, GE: 23.5 ± 4, HS: 19 ± 1).

3.5. Task and parameters

MEG data was acquired at a sampling rate of 1 kHz, with on-line band-pass filter of 0.10–330 Hz. Acquisition occurred in a single 20 min session of "resting state"; 10 min with eyes open looking to a cross on the screen followed by 10 min with eyes closed.

3.6. Removing artifacts

To correct the head position and the associated movement-related artifacts, a spatio-temporal signal space separation method (tSSS) with movement compensation (MC) was applied using the MaxFilter® software (Elekta Neuromag®, Elekta Oy, Helsinki, Finland). The use of tSSS is especially important for rejection of close-to-sensor artifacts.

After data reconstruction by signal space separation (referred as SSS), tSSS identifies artifacts by their correlated temporal behavior inside and outside the sensor helmet. The artifacts to be eliminated are thresholded by the quantitative level of this correlation determined by correlation limit of 0.95, and a correlation windows length of 10ms.

For each subject, artifact free epochs were then carefully selected by visual analysis Artifacts were typically due to (eye) movements, drowsiness or technical issues.

3.7. Used data

All the analysis were performed on 960 non-overlapping quasistationary segments (40 segments per subject) of 5000 ms free from eye or muscular artifacts, and epileptic activities (as, e.g., seizures or epileptic-like activity) and far (at least 20s) from recent epileptic discharges. The period of resting state with closed eyes was selected for the study. A downsampling to 500Hz was applied, thus obtaining segments of 2500 samples, as this has proven to be sufficient to detect clinically relevant differences in functional or effective connectivity in previous studies.

One important practical issue we would like to tackle here is that, in human MEG recording, not all types of magnetic sensors have the same sensitivity to deep brain sources. Magnetometers measure the overall magnitude of the magnetic field component approximately normal to the head surface; whereas planar gradiometers measure the difference of that field component at two adjacent locations. Describing MEG sensors in descending order of sensitivity to the depth of sources, magnetometers are most sensitive, followed by first-order axial gradiometers, second-order gradiometers and, finally, planar gradiometers [14]. Hence, planar gradiometers have maximum sensitivity to sources directly under them, i.e., superficial cortical sources [15], which makes them less sensitive to artifacts and distant disturbances, and therefore are suitable for studying this case, as these kinds of epilepsy have a neocortical origin. However, for the analysis, data from both the planar gradiometers and the magnetometers, was used.

4. Data analysis

4.1. Data preprocessing

In agreement with previous findings, surrogate data tests revealed that less than 4% of interdependencies between the spontaneous brain activities were nonlinear [16]. Thus, weighted brain networks were constructed by means of a definition of functional links based on Granger Causality (GC).

Application of GC requires that each time series is 'covariance stationary' (CS), i.e., that its mean and variance do not change over time. CS can be assessed in a rule-of-thumb way by examining the auto-correlation function. A non-CS time series will have an autocorrelation function that falls off slowly; a CS time series will have a sharply declining autocorrelation function. For this reason is that we take segments far enough from the spikes (at least 20s).

Prior to the causality analysis, we detrended the signals (subtracting the best-fitting line from each time series) and removed their temporal mean to provide a 'zero-mean' situation [17]. Granger causality analysis was performed to each segment of data (Anil Seth Toolbox [18]). The order of the autoregressive (AR) model was set to 4 according to the Bayesian Information Criterion (BIC) for our particular data [19].

4.2. Granger causality

As commented above, for two simultaneously measured signals, if one can predict the first signal better by incorporating the past information from the second signal than using only information from the first one, then the second signal can be called causal to the first one [5].The simplest way of quantifying this is by using univariate vs. bivariate linear regression models of a signal $x(t)$, to compare the forecast errors obtained incorporating (bivariate) or not (univariate) information from the past of $y(t)$.

For the univariate autoregressive model (AR), we have:

$$x(n) = \sum_{k=1}^{P} a_{x,k} x(n-k) + u_x(n)$$
$$y(n) = \sum_{k=1}^{P} a_{y,k} y(n-k) + u_y(n)$$

(1)

where a_{ij} are the model parameters (coefficients usually estimated by least square method), P is the order of the AR model and u_i, are the residuals associated to the model. Here, the prediction of each signal is performed only by its own past.

$$V_{X|\bar{X}} = \mathrm{var}(u_X)$$
$$V_{Y|\bar{Y}} = \mathrm{var}(u_Y)$$

(2)

Accordingly, for the bivariate AR:

$$x(n) = \sum_{k=1}^{P} a_{X|X,k} x(n-k) + \sum_{k=1}^{P} a_{X|Y,k} y(n-k) + u_{XY}(n)$$
$$y(n) = \sum_{k=1}^{P} a_{Y|X,k} x(n-k) + \sum_{k=1}^{P} a_{Y|Y,k} y(n-k) + u_{YX}(n)$$

(3)

where the residuals u_{XY} and u_{YX} now depend on the past values of both signals, and their variance is:

$$V_{X|\bar{X},\bar{Y}} = \mathrm{var}(u_{XY})$$
$$V_{Y|\bar{X},\bar{Y}} = \mathrm{var}(u_{YX})$$

(4)

where var(.) denote variance over time and $X \mid \overline{X}, \overline{Y}$ is the prediction of x(t) by the past samples of values of x(t) and y(t).

Therefore, Granger causality from y(t) to x(t) (predicting X from Y) is:

$$GC_{Y \rightarrow X} = \ln\left(\frac{V_{X \mid \overline{X}}}{V_{X \mid \overline{X},\overline{Y}}}\right) \tag{5}$$

GC ranges from 0 to infinity. The lower bound indicates that the incorporating information about the past of y(t) *does not* improve the prediction of x(t): $V_{X \mid \overline{X}} \approx V_{X \mid \overline{X},\overline{Y}}$. Accordingly, [4] is greater than 0, when the past of y(t) *does* improve the prediction of x(t): $V_{X \mid \overline{X}} > V_{X \mid \overline{X},\overline{Y}}$ (Y G-causes X)

As indicated in the Introduction, GC belongs to the category of asymmetric connectivity indexes; therefore, it assesses effective rather than functional connectivity. However, as defined from AR models it is a linear parametric method, so it is only sensitive to linear correlations and depends on the order (P) of the autoregressive. (See [20] for an extension of the GC concept to assess nonlinear interdependencies)

4.2.1. Significance of GC values

If we calculated the GC index [5] for all possible pair of sensors of the same kind (e.g. magnetometers, planar gradiometers along one axis and planar gradiometers along the two orthogonal axis) we get three connectivity matrixes, where each element $GC_{i \rightarrow j}$ measures the degree in which the signal in the sensor i Granger-causes that of the sensor j (i,j=1,..,102). However, it is necessary to determine whether the value of each given index is due to real causal dependence between the corresponding two sensors or rather it is not zero due to statistical fluctuations in the estimation of variance of the forecasting. This task can be easily accomplished because it is known that time-domain GC interaction is significant if the coefficients a_{ij} are jointly significantly different from zero. This can be established via an F-test on the null hypothesis that A_{ij} are zero [6].

These have to be corrected for multiple comparisons, which we do here by applying the well-known 'false discovery rate' (FDR) method [21–23] at a desired significance threshold of 0.05. In all the cases where the (corrected) test failed to reject the null hypothesis, the corresponding GC index is set to zero.

Moreover, recent results show that correlations between magnetic fields sensors located at a distance less than 4 cm cannot distinguish between spontaneous activities of epileptic patients and control subjects [24]. To reduce the influence of these spurious correlations between MEG signals, we have excluded the nearest sensors (separated less than 4 cm) from the computation of Granger causality values.

The final effective connectivity matrixes so obtained can be interpreted as the adjacency matrix of a directed weighted network. Hence, network analysis methods derived from graph theory

[25] could be applied to assess the most significant features of the brain connectivity networks in the groups of subjects described before (i.e. GE, FE and HS), during the resting state task with closed eyes [26,27]. And from that, study their differences.

4.3. Network parameters

To characterize the network structure of brain activity of each group of subjects, we evaluated a list of measures for directed weighted graphs [28]. In this approach, MEG sensors were considered as vertices (nodes) and the GC values between sensors as edge weights (links). The edge weight represents the strength of the connection between the vertices.

Here some notation is explained (see [25] for details):

- N is the set of all nodes in the network, and n is the number of nodes.

- L is the set of all links in the network, and l is number of links.

- (i, j) is a link between nodes i and j, where i,j $\in$ N.

- Links (i, j) are associated with connection weights w_{ij}.

- a_{ij} is the connection status between i and j: $a_{ij} = 1$ when link (i, j) exists (when i and j are neighbors); $a_{ij} = 0$ otherwise ($a_{ii} = 0$ for all i).

- We compute the number of links as $l = \sum_{i,j \in N} a_{ij}$ (to avoid ambiguity with directed links we count each undirected link twice, as a_{ij} and as a_{ji}).

- The sum of all weights in the network is l^w, and it is computed as $l^w = \sum_{i,j \in N} w_{ij}$. Henceforth, we assume that weights are normalized, such that $0 \leq w_{ij} \leq 1$ for all i and j.

We focused on the following global parameters, to be explained henceforth: the average degree (section 4.3.1), strength (section 4.3.2) and two measures of segregation, namely the clustering coefficient (section 4.3.3) and modularity (section 4.3.4).

4.3.1. Degree

The degree (D) of a node is the number of links connected to it. In directed weighted networks, we distinguish between the 'in degree', which is the number of links that arrive to the node, and the 'out degree', which is the number of links that go out from the node.

- (Directed) in-degree of i, $k^{in}_i = \sum_{j \in N} a_{ji}$

- (Directed) out-degree of i, $k^{out}_i = \sum_{j \in N} a_{ij}$

The global degree of a network is the average of all its nodes' degree. The mean network degree is most commonly used as a measure of density, or the total "wiring cost" of the network.

4.3.2. Strength

The weighted variant of the degree, sometimes termed the *strength*, is defined as the sum of all neighboring link weights.

4.3.3. Clustering coefficient

The clustering coefficient (C) describes the likelihood that neighbors of a vertex are also connected. It quantifies the tendency of network elements to form local clusters. We used the directed and weighted equivalent of this measure to characterize local clustering [29]:

$$C^{\rightarrow} = \frac{1}{n} \sum_{i \in N} \frac{t_i^{\rightarrow}}{\left(k_i^{out} + k_i^{in}\right)\left(k_i^{out} + k_i^{in} - 1\right) - 2 \sum_{j \in N} a_{ij} a_{ji}} \tag{6}$$

Here and in the following equation, the arrow next to the indexes denotes that they are calculated for directed networks. However, for the sake of clarity in the text, we will omit this arrow in the name of the indexes henceforth.

4.3.4. Modularity

Modularity (Q) quantifies how a network can be optimally divided in subgroups or modules. We used a modification for directed weighted networks by [30]

$$Q^{\rightarrow} = \frac{1}{l} \sum_{i,j \in N} \left[a_{ij} - \frac{k_i^{out} k_j^{in}}{l} \right] \delta_{m_i m_j} \tag{7}$$

Roughly speaking, the greater the value of Q, the more modular a network is, i.e., the greater the density of within-cluster connections as compared to the between-cluster ones.

4.4. Statistical tests

4.4.1. Between groups comparisons

We performed a Kruskal Wallis test to compare network parameters from the three groups (FE, GE, HS). This test compares the medians of the samples in each group, and returns the p value for the rejection of the null hypothesis that all samples are drawn from the same population (or equivalently, from different populations with the same distribution). The Kruskal-Wallis test is a nonparametric version of the classical one-way ANOVA, and an extension of the Wilcoxon rank sum test to more than two groups.

If the p value is close zero, this suggests that at least one sample median is significantly different from the others. Here, we took p<0.05 as the critical value to determine whether the null hypothesis can be rejected.

4.4.2. Post-hoc between (two) groups comparisons

In those cases where the Kruskall-Wallis to check was significant, we further analyzed pairwise difference between any two groups by means of a two-sided rank sum test (Wilcoxon test),

test the null hypothesis that the network parameters obtained for each group of subjects are independent samples from identical continuous distributions with equal medians, against the alternative that they do not have equal medians. This test is equivalent to a Mann-Whitney U-test. Differences were again considered significant if p<0.05.

5. Results

Differences in the global network parameters between the three groups (FE, GE and HS):

5.1. Differences among the planar gradiometer networks

The interdependence matrixes obtained from the planar gradiometers were sparse, i.e., they presented only a few significant GC values (effective links) between the corresponding neocortical sources. Differences among groups for the planar gradiometers were found in modularity (see figure 1).

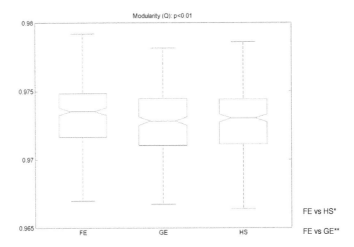

Figure 1. Modularity Q (equation (7)) of the brain networks of planar gradiometers for the healthy subjects (HS), and patients with either focal (FE) or global epilepsy (GE). The Kruskal Wallis tests for global differences among the three groups was highly significant (p<0.01). Asterisks denote differences between any two groups; *: p<0.05; * p<0.01. The boxplots are median (red line), and the 25% and 75% percentiles (blue box), whereas the whiskers indicates the maximum and minimum of each group.

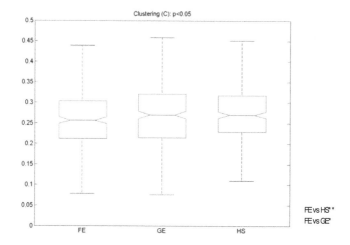

Figure 2. Clustering coefficient C (equation (6)) for the networks of magnetometers. Global differences (Kruskal Wallis test) were significant at the p<0.01 level. Group notation, boxplots, whiskers and differences between two groups as in figure 1.

Patients suffering from frontal focal epilepsy, present a higher value of Q as compared to those suffering from generalized epilepsy and healthy subjects. Differences in magnetometers

5.2. Between-group differences in brain networks recorded from magnetometers

Differences in network parameters for magnetometers were found in cluster coefficient (figure 2), degree (figure 3), strength (figure 4) and number of clusters (figure 5).

As can be seen from figure 2, the FE group presents a lower value of C than those from the GE and the HS group.

Also, for the average degree D (figure 3) patients from the FE group, present a higher value of global network degree as compared to GE patients and healthy controls.

Moreover, for the average strength S (figure 4), FE patients showed the highest values of the index as compared to GE patients and healthy controls.

Finally, for the number of clusters (figure 5) healthy subjects present a lower number of clusters as compared to both group of epileptic.

6. Discussion

The assessment of functional brain networks from multivariate fMRI, EEG or MEG data has become a very popular line of research nowadays [25,31]. This is most likely because the

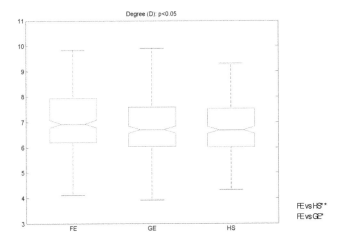

Figure 3. Average degree D for the networks of magnetometers. Global differences (Kruskal Wallis test) were significant at the p<0.05 level. Group notation, boxplots, whiskers and differences between two groups are as in previous figures.

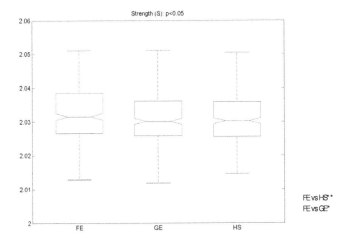

Figure 4. Average strength (S) for the networks of magnetometers. Global differences (Kruskal Wallis test) were significant at the p<0.05 level. Group notation, boxplots, whiskers and differences between two groups as in previous figures.

parameters derived from this approach are relatively easy to calculate and interpret in neurophysiological terms. In fact, one only needs, on the one hand, a measure of functional or

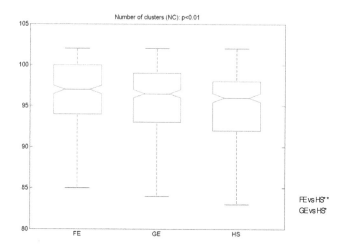

Figure 5. Average number of clusters in the networks of magnetometers. Global differences (Kruskal Wallis test) were significant at the p<0.01 level. Group notation, boxplots, whiskers and differences between two groups as in previous figures.

effective connectivity between any two signals and, on the other, a way of estimating the significance of such a measure. Once you are equipped with these two tools, the characterization of the corresponding brain network is only a few calculations ahead.

Yet even these apparently straightforward steps (e.g., estimation of bivariate connectivity index and their significance) are deceptively simple, and their careless, mechanical application may result in misleading results and/or false conclusions. Common sources of error are the misuse of a given connectivity index, failing to assess its significance in a proper way or not taking into account what the data we have recorded are actually measuring. This latter issue is specially significant when dealing with extra-cranially recorded signals (whether EEG or MEG data), in which it is well-known that signals in different sensors are often measuring the activity of the same deep brain source, this resulting in a statistically significant relationship between these signals that has very few (if any) to do with the existence of connectivity between the sensors.

This important question can be tackled in different ways. One obvious attempt consists in trying to reconstruct, from the recorded data, the neurological sources of activity before applying the network connectivity approach. But the so-called inverse problem of source reconstruction is known to be ill-posed, in the sense that it is underdetermined, as the number of sources is much larger than that of the measures, and has not a single solution. Another possibility includes the use of carefully devised indexes [32], which are robust against common source effects but which, unfortunately, are not without their own particular problems [33]. In this work, we have dealt with the question in a different way, by taking advantage of the complementary information provided by two kinds of sensors (magnetometers and planar gradiometers) in a modern MEG recording device. The key idea consists in the fact that whereas magnetometers are sensitive to all sources (whether cortical or deep ones) in the direction normal to the head surface where they record, gradiometers are only sensitive to cortical sources *right behind* the recorded surface [14], and therefore unlikely to be affected by the common source problem. Thus, comparing the results from the magnetometers and the planar gradiometers recorded simultaneously from the same subject, we may get insight into the possible effect that common sources has on the functional brain network assessed by the former sensors, which are by far the most common sensors used in MEG literature.

Here, we have applied this approach to study brain networks of effective connectivity from planar gradiometers and magnetometers recorded during rest with closed eyes in three groups of subjects, one of healthy controls and two of patients suffering from different kinds of epilepsy: generalized and frontal focal. The connectivity index used was the GC index, whose significant was assessed by a careful combination of F-test estimation and FDR statistical test to deal with the multiple comparison problem. And we think we might rightly conclude that the results obtained justify our use of what we may call this *multi-sensor approach*. Indeed, thanks to it, two important questions have come out. First, if we were to analyze the data from the magnetometers alone, we would have come to the conclusions that the functional networks from the three groups are different in a number of parameters, whereas these networks, when only the cortical sources are recorded, do not present differences among the three groups in any of these parameters. Second, networks of cortical sources do present differences in modularity between healthy and epileptic groups, as well as between the two epileptic patients.

Thus, by analyzing the information provided by the combined use of both sensors, we have a greater insight into the brain networks of the three groups (and the differences among them). The information from the planar gradiometers suggests that connectivity between neocortical sources is sparse, and the corresponding networks are only weakly modular (low Q), but the intra-cluster connectivity of the epileptic groups are greater than that of healthy subjects, with the FE group in turn being significantly more modular than the GE group. This result is very interesting, as it is well-known that the greater the intra-cluster connectivity, the easier it is for a network to become fully synchronized [34]. Thus, it would indicate that in both types of epilepsy, the network of neocortical sources is more prone to become (pathologically) synchronized that in normal subjects.

When we review the information from the magnetometers, we can get information about deeper brain sources. The first interesting result is that the networks constructed from magnetometers are more densely connected that those from the gradiometers. Besides, these networks are scarcely modular in any of the groups (as the number of clusters in Figure 5 is close to the number of sensors) and present a higher number of (stronger) links (higher C, D and S as shown in figures 2, 3 and 4, respectively) in the epileptic groups as compared to healthy subjects. Unfortunately, it is difficult to interpret these results simply in terms of the corresponding connectivity between deep sources, as the possibility of the same source being recorded in different magnetometers cannot be ruled out. Yet rather than whether these results are a consequence of more active deep sources or more interconnected ones, what is really important is the fact that network theory as applied to MEG data is able to disclose changes in neurological activity of epileptic subjects as compared to healthy subjects even when no epileptogenic activity is apparent in the raw data.

6.1. Future work

The results presented above are certainly interesting, not only because of their methodological and neurological implications, but also because they pave the way for future studies in the same line. One obvious question to further investigate from these data is whether the between-groups differences found in various global parameters in both planar gradiometers and magnetometers can be explored in terms of their (possibly local) origin. Namely, whether they are due to local differences between the corresponding networks, which are detected by these global parameters but can be also characterized topologically. Indeed, it is tempting to hypothesize that the FE group, whose epilepsy has a focal origin, presents differences with both the GE and the HS group precisely in the frontal sensors. Another important question that we should elucidate is whether differences are present at all the frequencies of the signal or are rather constrained to a certain frequency band (as found in former works [26]), but detected here by the GC index, which operates on the broadband signal in the time domain. One last issue of practical interest that we are currently studying is the possible usefulness of the differences in network connectivity patterns to assist in the classification (diagnosis) of recorded subjects using machine learning algorithms. This latter application is potentially very important from the clinical point of view. Additionally, it would also allow circumventing the problem of determining if the patterns of GC index (or any other connectivity index for that matter) are due to true connectivity or are the result of volume conduction of deep brain sources, which are reflected in many sensors at the same time. As long as these patterns are different in each group, they would be useful to detect deviations from healthy condition. Here also, the fact that the information from the two type of magnetic sensors available (magnetometers and planar gradiometers) is not redundant but complementary, speaks clearly in favor of analyzing both sensors at the same time, whenever possible.

We hope that this line of research will continue to provide further insight into the pattern of connectivity networks in health and disease and its possible application as an additional tool for diagnostic purposes in different neurologic pathologies.

Acknowledgements

Guiomar Niso, Ernesto Pereda and Francisco del Pozo acknowledge the financial support of the Spanish Ministry of Economy and Competitiveness through the grants TEC2012-38453-CO4-01 and -03. Fernando Maestú, María Gudín and Sira Carrasco acknowledge the financial support of the Castilla La Mancha Sanitary System through grant PS09/00450. Guiomar Niso has also received the financial support of the Spanish Ministry of Education and Science through the FPU grant AP2008-02383.

Author details

Guiomar Niso[1*], Ernesto Pereda[2], Fernando Maestú[1], María Gudín[3], Sira Carrasco[3] and Francisco del-Pozo[1]

*Address all correspondence to: guiomar.niso@ctb.upm.es

1 Center for Biomedical Technology, Technical University of Madrid, Madrid, Spain

2 Electrical Engineering and Bioengineering Group, Dept. of Basic Physics, University of La Laguna, Tenerife, Spain

3 Ciudad Real Universitary Hospital, Ciudad Real, Spain

References

[1] Buzsaki G. Rhythms of the Brain. Oxford University Press; 2006 Oct 26;

[2] Bressler SL. Large-scale cortical networks and cognition. Brain Research. Brain Research Reviews. 1995 Mar;20(3):288–304.

[3] Varela F, Lachaux J, Rodriguez E, Martinerie J. The brainweb: phase synchronization and large-scale integration", Nature Review Neuroscience 2001, 2(4):229-39.

[4] Friston KJ. Functional and effective connectivity in neuroimaging: A synthesis. Human Brain Mapping. 1994 Oct 13;2(1-2):56–78.

[5] Wiener N. The Theory of Prediction. In: Beckenbach EF, editor. Modern mathematics for the engineer. New York: McGraw-Hill; 1956. p. 165 – 190.

[6] Granger C. Investigating causal relations by econometric models and cross-spectral methods. Econometrica: Journal of the Econometric Society. 1969;37(3):424–38.

[7] Pereda E, Quiroga RQ, Bhattacharya J, Quian Quiroga R. Nonlinear multivariate analysis of neurophysiological signals. Progress in Neurobiology. 2005;77(1-2):1–37.

[8] Freiwald W, Valdes P, Bosch J, Biscay R, Jimenez JC, Rodriguez LM, et al. Testing non-linearity and directedness of interactions between neural groups in the macaque inferotemporal cortex. Journal of Neuroscience Methods. 1999 Dec 15;94(1):105–19.

[9] Bernasconi C, Von Stein A, Chiang C, König P. Bi-directional interactions between visual areas in the awake behaving cat. Neuroreport. 2000 Mar 20;11(4):689–92.

[10] Salazar RF, König P, Kayser C. Directed interactions between visual areas and their role in processing image structure and expectancy. The European Journal of Neuroscience. 2004 Sep;20(5):1391–401.

[11] Brovelli A, Ding M, Ledberg A, Chen Y, Nakamura R, Bressler SL. Beta oscillations in a large-scale sensorimotor cortical network: directional influences revealed by Granger causality. Proceedings of the National Academy of Sciences of the United States of America. 2004 Jun 29;101(26):9849–54.

[12] Hesse W, Möller E, Arnold M, Schack B. The use of time-variant EEG Granger causality for inspecting directed interdependencies of neural assemblies. Journal of Neuroscience Methods. 2003 Mar;124(1):27–44.

[13] Bressler SL. AKS. Wiener–Granger Causality: A well established methodology. NeuroImage. 2011, 15;58(2):323-9

[14] Hansen P, Kringelbach M, Salmelin R. MEG An Introduction to methods. Oxford University Press. 2010. p. 448.

[15] Hämäläinen MS. Functional localization based on measurements with a whole-head magnetometer system. Brain Topography. Springer New York; 1995;7(4):283–9.

[16] Stam CJ, Breakspear M, Van Cappellen van Walsum A-M, Van Dijk BW. Nonlinear synchronization in EEG and whole-head MEG recordings of healthy subjects. Human Brain Mapping. 2003 Jun;19(2):63–78.

[17] Ding M, Bressler SL, Yang W, Liang H. Short-window spectral analysis of cortical event-related potentials by adaptive multivariate autoregressive modeling: data pre-processing, model validation, and variability assessment. Biological Cybernetics. Springer; 2000 Jul;83(1):35–45.

[18] Seth AK. A MATLAB toolbox for Granger causal connectivity analysis. Journal of Neuroscience Methods. Elsevier B.V.; 2010 Feb 15;186(2):262–73.

[19] Schwarz G. Estimating the dimension of a model. The Annals of Statistics. 1978;6(2): 461–4.

[20] Ancona N, Marinazzo D, Stramaglia S. Radial basis function approach to nonlinear Granger causality of time series. Physical Review E. 2004 Nov;70(5):056221.

[21] Benjamini Y, Hochberg Y. Controlling the false discovery rate: a practical and powerful approach to multiple testing. Journal of the Royal Statistical Society. Series B. 1995; 57:289-300

[22] Benjamini Y, Yekutieli D. The control of the false discovery rate in multiple testing under dependency. Annals of Statistics. 2001;29(4):1165–88.

[23] Genovese CR, Lazar N a, Nichols T. Thresholding of statistical maps in functional neuroimaging using the false discovery rate. NeuroImage. 2002 Apr;15(4):870–8.

[24] Garcia Dominguez L, Wennberg R a, Gaetz W, Cheyne D, Snead OC, Perez Velazquez JL. Enhanced synchrony in epileptiform activity? Local versus distant phase synchronization in generalized seizures. The Journal of Neuroscience. 2005 Aug 31;25(35):8077–84.

[25] Rubinov M, Sporns O. Complex network measures of brain connectivity: uses and interpretations. NeuroImage. 2010;52(3):1059–69.

[26] Chavez M, Valencia M, Navarro V, Latora V, Martinerie J. Functional Modularity of Background Activities in Normal and Epileptic Brain Networks. Physical Review Letters. 2010;104(11):1–4.

[27] Van Dellen E, Douw L, Hillebrand A, Ris-Hilgersom IHM, Schoonheim MM, Baayen JC, et al. MEG Network Differences between Low- and High-Grade Glioma Related to Epilepsy and Cognition. PloS one. 2012 Jan;7(11):e50122.

[28] Boccaletti S, Latora V, Moreno Y, Chavez M, Hwang D. Complex networks: Structure and dynamics. Physics Reports. 2006 Feb;424(4-5):175–308.

[29] Fagiolo G. Clustering in complex directed networks. Physical Review E. 2007; 76(2): 026107

[30] Leicht E, Newman M. Community structure in directed networks. Physical Review Letters. 2008;1–5.

[31] Stam CJ, Van Straaten ECW. The organization of physiological brain networks. Clinical Neurophysiology. 2012 Jun;123(6):1067–87.

[32] Stam CJ, Nolte G, Daffertshofer A. Phase lag index: assessment of functional connectivity from multi channel EEG and MEG with diminished bias from common sources. Human Brain Mapping. 2007 Nov;28(11):1178–93.

[33] Vinck M, Oostenveld R, Van Wingerden M, Battaglia F, Pennartz CM a. An improved index of phase-synchronization for electrophysiological data in the presence of volume-conduction, noise and sample-size bias. NeuroImage. 2011 Apr 15;55(4): 1548–65.

[34] Balanov A, Janson N, Postnov D, Sosnovtseva O. Synchronization: From Simple to Complex. Berlin: Springer Series in Synergetics, Springer; 2009.

Chapter 4

Optimized Signal Separation for 3D-Polarized Light Imaging

Jürgen Dammers, Lukas Breuer, Giuseppe Tabbì and Markus Axer

Additional information is available at the end of the chapter

1. Introduction

1.1. Anatomical connectivity mapping

"Why should we bother about connectivity in the age of functional imaging, at a time when magnets of ever increasing strength promise to detect the location of even the faintest thought? Isn't it enough to locate cortical areas engaged in deception, introspection, empathy? Do we really have to worry about their connections? The answer is "yes". In the case of the nervous system, the unit of relational architecture that allows the whole to exceed the sum of the parts is known as large-scale network. Its elucidation requires an elaborate understanding of connectivity patterns" [1]. Despite considerable advances in experimental techniques and in our understanding of animal anatomy over the last decades, the real connectivity of the human brain has essentially remained a mystery. It is the human brain's multiscale topology that poses a particular challenge to any neuroimaging technique and prevented the neuroscientists from unraveling the connectome so far.

However, it is also the brain's architecture that allows different morphological entities to be defined at different scales depending on the spatial resolution provided by the available neuroimaging techniques and the scientific objectives. Consequently, a comprehensive description of neuronal networks and their intricate fiber connections requires a multimodal approach based on complementary imaging techniques targeting different levels of organization (microscale, mesoscale, and macroscale) [2,3].

MR-based diffusion imaging is the most frequently used method to visualize fiber pathways in both the living and the postmortem human brain (for a comprehensive introduction to the field cf. [4,5]). Diffusion imaging contributes to the understanding of the macroscopic connectivity (i.e., at the millimeter scale) in the living brain, while postmortem studies already explore the upper mesoscale (i.e., the sub-millimeter scale). Hence, not surprisingly, diffusion imaging is of great appeal to neuroscientists as a method for the visualization of connectivity patterns in both clinical and basic research. However, complex fiber networks and small fiber tracts are difficult to be disentangled reliably at present. Furthermore, the termination of fields of pathways emanating from cortical areas no larger than a few millimeters in size cannot be demonstrated with the required precision.

Conversely, microscopic techniques generate data sets of impressing neuroanatomical detail, but they are limited to small sample sizes (i.e., small areas of interest in a small number of subjects) of postmortem tissue. This substantially restricts their predictive power. In the recent years, anatomical connections in the human postmortem brains were studied with dissection techniques [6,7], in myelin stained sections of adult human brains [8], or of immature brains taking advantage of heterochronic myelination of different fiber tracts during pre- and early postnatal development [9], in lesioned brains using various techniques for staining degenerating fibers [10,11], and using tract-tracing methods for discovering local connections [12,13]. These studies have enriched our knowledge about human brain fiber tracts, but all of them suffer from severe restrictions if the 3D courses of fiber pathways are to be mapped in the adult human brain. In contrast to studies in animals, the tight packing of different fiber tracts in the white substance, and the lack of specific tracers for in vitro tracking of long distance fibers made comprehensive fiber tract mapping impossible in the adult human brain [14].

1.2. 3D-polarized light imaging (3D-PLI)

Recently, a neuroimaging technique referred to as *3D-polarized light imaging (3D-PLI)* has been introduced that has opened up new avenues to study human brain regions with complex fiber architecture as well as small cortical fibers at the micrometer level [15–17]. This technique is applicable to microtome sections of postmortem brains and utilizes the optically birefringence of nerve fibers, which is induced by the optical anisotropy of the myelin sheaths surrounding axons [18–20]. 3D-PLI provides a three-dimensional description of the anatomical connectivity in form of a vector field indicating the prevailing fiber orientation per voxel. Depending on the used imaging setup and the section thickness the acquirable spatial resolution is 1.6 – 100 μm. Hence, the method bridges the microscopic and the macroscopic description of the anatomical connectivity of the human brain.

The birefringence of brain tissue is measured by passing linearly polarized light through histological brain sections and by detecting local changes in the polarization state of light using a polarimeter setup (Figure 1a-b). The polarimeter is equipped with a pair of crossed polarizers, a tilting specimen stage, a quarter-wave retarder, an LED light source (with a narrow-band green wavelength spectrum), and a charge-coupled device (CCD) camera. By rotating the optical devices simultaneously around the stationary brain section and by imaging the sample at discrete rotation angles ρ, a sinusoidal variation of the measured light intensity (i.e., the light intensity profile) is observed for each image pixel (Figure 1c). The individual course of a light intensity profile essentially depends on the locally prevailing 3D fiber orientation described by an orientation unit vector which is defined by the in-section direction angle φ and the out-of-section inclination angle α. Basic principles of optics (Snell's law and Huygens-Fresnel principle) and the Jones calculus [21] mathematically link the measured light intensity profile I to the fiber orientation via

$$I = \frac{I_0}{2} \cdot [1 + sin(2\rho - 2\varphi) \cdot sin\delta], \qquad (1)$$

with $\delta \approx 2\pi \cdot \frac{d \cdot \Delta n}{\lambda} \cdot cos^2\alpha$.

The amplitude of the profile quantifies the phase retardation δ induced to the light wave by the myelin. This phase retardation is a function of the light wavelength λ, the section thickness d, the birefringence Δn of the myelin, and the inclination angle α. The transmittance I_0 denotes the intensity of the incident light modified by local extinction effects. While ρ is the azimuth angle of the transmission axis of the first polarizer, φ represents the projection of the fiber axis onto the section plane with respect to the starting angle of the polarimeter. As a consequence, the fundamental data structure gained by 3D-PLI is a 3D vector field description of fibers and fiber tract orientations – the basis for subsequent tractography and fiber modeling.

For estimating the sinusoidal profile of the 3D-PLI signal Discrete Fourier Analysis (DFA) can be used to deduce I from Equation (1):

$$I = a_0 + a_1 \cdot sin(2\rho) + b_1 \cdot cos(2\rho) \qquad (2)$$

with $a_0 = \frac{I_0}{2}$, $a_1 = \frac{I_0}{2} \cdot sin(\delta) \cdot cos(2\varphi)$, $b_1 = \frac{I_0}{2} \cdot sin(\delta) \cdot sin(2\varphi)$.

1.3. Relevance and restoration of the light intensity profile

In 3D-PLI, the light intensity profile (cf. Figure 1) represents a crucial data set in terms of fiber orientation determination, since peak position and signal amplitude of the profile are directly related to the in-section direction and out-of-section inclination of the fiber orientation, respectively. A precise and undisturbed recording of the light intensity passing through a microtome section is therefore mandatory for the reliable reconstruction of high-resolution fiber tracts. The signal quality is however influenced by several conditions. Thermal effects and electrical noise in both the light source and the CCD-electronics deteriorate the PLI signal characteristics at each image pixel. Filter inhomogeneities of the polarizers or retarder may also manipulate the intensity profile. Therefore, a standardized image calibration technique using flat fields is usually applied to all raw images prior to analysis to compensate pixel-wise for inhomogeneities across the field-of-view [22]. Depending on the section thickness the pixel-by-pixel intensity is also influenced by the scatter properties of the investigated object. Another possible source of artifacts is dust on the polarizer. Although the polarimeter should be operated in a shielded construction to prevent for external light and dust particles, dust cannot completely be avoided. As a result of the rotation of the polarizer dust particles will deteriorate the measured light intensity only once within a half circle, if and only if they are located on the rotating system (cf. Figure 1). Hence, the measured intensity at the CCD array is a linear mixture of different light sources.

Recently, signal enhancement and restoration techniques for PLI images utilizing independent component analysis (ICA) have been introduced [22,23]. As a result, component maps corresponding to gray and white matter structures as well as noise and artifacts can be identified automatically using statistical analysis tools [23]. Remarkably, even in the presence of dust on the polarimeter ICA can effectively restore the original sinusoidal signal (Figure 2). After ICA filtering the noise and artifacts are removed and the sinusoidal nature of the PLI signal is restored (Figure 2).

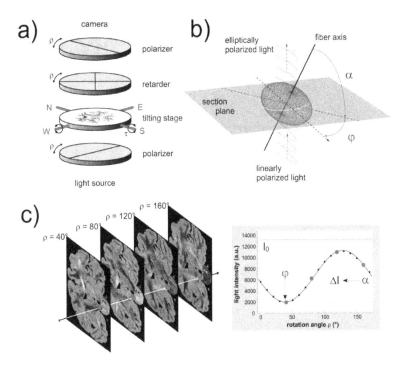

Figure 1. Polarimetry at a glance. (a) Scheme of the rotating polarimeter with tilting stage (N-North, W-West, E-East, S-South). (b) Scheme of the optical fiber model. The refractive index of a negative uniaxially birefringent medium, such as a myelinated axon, is described by an elliptically shaped oblate surface, the indicatrix (gray mesh). A beam of linearly polarized light (blue trace) interacts locally with the myelin sheath of a single axon (black line) and becomes elliptically polarized. (c) A typical 3D-PLI raw image data set consists of 18 images corresponding to equidistant rotation angles between 0° and 170°. Here, a selection of four images of a coronal section is shown, while the sketched arrow indicates one representative pixel. To obtain the fiber orientation, the measured light intensities are studied pixel-wise as a function of discrete rotation angles. The derived physical model provides a precise mathematical description of the measurement (continuous black line) and relates the sine phase to the direction angle φ and the amplitude to the inclination angle α. The highlighted data points correspond to the selected images.

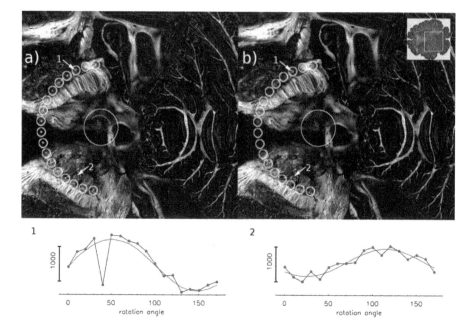

Figure 2. In (a) multiple artifacts including dust contamination are present. The trajectory of a dust particle is high-lighted by the signal power inside the white circles along all rotation angles. After ICA filtering (b) the signal deroga-tion is greatly removed. At the bottom, PLI raw signals (black) are shown together with corresponding signals after artifact rejection (red). The signals were extracted from the two locations as indicated by the red dots. In comparison to the PLI raw data ICA obviously removed the signal derogation and is capable of restoring the original sinusoidal signal in case of dust (signal #1) or noise (signal #2) contaminations.

2. A new concept for optimal signal decomposition in polarized light imaging

Although blind source separation methods are successfully applied for signal separation in all kinds of neuroimaging modalities [24–29] two major problems remain: i) the method applied must be selected carefully and the separation strategy (i.e., the internal cost function) of the applied method should be optimal for the type of data. This however, is one of the reasons why many different ICA algorithms co-exist. ii) Assuming the measured signals are adequately separated into the underlying source signals (i.e., signal of interest and non-interest), identi-fication of the signal of interest should be performed user independently; preferably in an automatic fashion. For the latter, significant effort has to be invested in order to identify components of interest automatically from data recorded utilizing different neuroimaging techniques [29–33]. In contrast to many other ICA applications, the great advantage in PLI signal decomposition is that all profiles of the basis vectors that correspond to the signal of interest must show a sinusoidal waveform [16,22]. Since these waveforms can only vary in amplitude and phase, an automatic extraction of the signal components can be achieved utilizing this property as demonstrated in [23].

Alternatively, it has been demonstrated that by incorporating prior knowledge, i.e., by imposing temporal or spatial constraints for the source separation task, decomposition can be effectively improved [34–37]. Hesse and James [38], for example, showed that using different types of spatial constraints ICA can be trained to *i)* identify ocular artifacts automatically and *ii)* to detect and trace ictal activity. Liu and colleagues recently presented a reference based ICA concept to successfully target a specific genetic variation [36] in real and simulated data sets. For the investigation of signal detection in the imaging system of the retina in cats Barriga and colleagues introduced a constrained ICA algorithm which increases the detection of responses to visual stimuli in cats even for low levels of signal-to-noise ratio [37]. In the next section the basic principle of ICA is described shortly. For a more detailed review, we refer to [39,40].

2.1. A short introduction to independent component analysis (ICA)

For 3D-PLI a linear superposition of light at the CCD camera is assumed, where each elementary signal component refers to a distinct region in space. By applying independent component analysis (ICA) to a set of polarized light images (here a stack of 18 images at different rotation angles is used) the decomposition of the data results in spatially independent components (often called feature or basis vectors) yielding maximally (i.e., statistically) independent spatial component maps.

Let $\mathbf{X}=(X_1, X_2, \ldots, X_N)^T$ be the N-dimensional measured PLI signal mixture, where each X_i is one image mixture (flatted to a one-dimensional image vector with M pixels) detected at a corresponding rotation angle ρ. In spatial ICA $\mathbf{X}$ is considered to be a $N \times M$ matrix (as opposed to temporal ICA, where the dimension of the matrix is transposed), with M = number of pixels included in the analysis and N = number of rotation angles reflecting N different instances of the signal. The contribution of each source image varies N times over the angles ρ. Similarly, $\mathbf{S}=(S_1, S_2, \ldots, S_N)^T$ represents the N-dimensional true source signals. Hence, the linear relationship of mixed sources can be expressed as follows:

$$\mathbf{X}=\mathbf{AS} \tag{3}$$

with $\mathbf{A}$ being the unknown mixing matrix of dimension $N \times N$. The key problem in ICA is to find an unmixing matrix $\mathbf{W}$ (similar to a pseudo-inverse $\mathbf{A}^{-1}$, with $\mathbf{W} \approx \mathbf{A}^{-1}$) while imposing that the sources in $\mathbf{S}$ are statistically independent, that is:

$$\mathbf{C}=\mathbf{WX}. \tag{4}$$

Within ICA the N-dimensional data array $\mathbf{X}$ is transformed into an N-dimensional component space $\mathbf{C}$, where each of the spatial component maps carries a minimum amount of mutual information and thus is maximally independent. These independent components (or spatial maps) are stored in the rows of $\mathbf{C}$, while in the columns of $\mathbf{W}^{-1}$ the associated spatially independent "temporal" profiles (i.e., the contrast changing function along the rotation angle, the basis vector) are stored.

Signal restoration, i.e. the cleaning process, is performed by zeroing columns in $\mathbf{W}^{-1}$ which reflect signal contributions from unwanted (e.g. artifact) sources. This is identical to zeroing rows in $\mathbf{C}$, where the independent component maps of interest are stored in $\mathbf{C}'$. The cleaning of measured data is performed by back transformation of $\mathbf{C}'$, which results in a new set of PLI data $\mathbf{X}'$.

$$\mathbf{X}' = \overset{\wedge}{\mathbf{A}} \cdot \mathbf{C}' \tag{5}$$

with $\mathbf{W}^{-1} = \overset{\wedge}{\mathbf{A}}$.

2.2. Constrained ICA for polarized light imaging (cICAP)

Signal separation in constrained ICA is based on incorporating prior knowledge about the underlying signals. In the study of Barriga and colleagues [37], *a priori* information is incorporated into one column of the estimated mixing matrix of the spatial decomposition via an off-on constraint, meaning that the visual response signal used in the study has to follow the stimulus signal. For this, the authors filled one column of the mixing matrix with ones for the time of the stimulation, while zero values reflect off-stimulation. Similar to the concept introduced by Barriga and colleagues in 2011, it is possible to incorporate the *a priori* information from 3D-PLI, but with the major difference that for birefringent signals an analytical expression exists to model the expected signal of interest, which only differs in amplitude and phase. Therefore, a new algorithm motivated by the results described in [23] has been developed, where signal separation and the identification of the underlying 3D-PLI source signals are combined into one method. The new algorithm (referred to as *constrained ICA for polarized light imaging, cICAP*) is based on a modified version of the Infomax principle [41] by means of incorporating prior information to the cost function of Infomax; this is similar to the work reported in [34,37]. In cICAP a theoretically expected function $f_i(u_\rho)$ is implemented into the Infomax cost function to control for the results of the decomposition. Recall that if the i-th column in $\mathbf{A}$ has a sinusoidal profile, the corresponding component map in $\mathbf{C}$ represents a signal of interest (cf. Equation (4-5)). The expected function $f_i(u_\rho)$ can be derived from Equation (2), where the parameters a_0, a_1 and b_1 are fitted involving all rotation angles ρ [16].

Starting from Equation (4) the natural-gradient version in Infomax is used to update the weight matrix $\mathbf{W}$ during the ICA learning procedure [42,43]:

$$\Delta\mathbf{W} = \left[\mathbf{I} + (1 - 2\mathbf{y})\mathbf{C}^{*T}\right]\mathbf{W} \tag{6}$$

with $\mathbf{y} = 1/\left(1 + e^{-\mathbf{C}^*}\right)$.

In Equation (6) $\mathbf{I}$ and   denote the identity matrix and the learning rate, respectively, as it is used in the standard Infomax algorithm [41]. $\mathbf{C}^*$ denotes the intermediate component matrix which is identical to $\mathbf{C}$ when the learning procedure is finished. In common with the approach of [37], the mixing matrix $\hat{\mathbf{A}}$ is estimated by $\hat{\mathbf{A}} := (\mathbf{P} \cdot \mathbf{W})^{-1}$, with $\mathbf{P}$ being the sphering matrix of the decorrelation process within Infomax. By incorporating the *a priori* information at each iteration step, $\hat{\mathbf{A}}$ is updated by:

$$\hat{\mathbf{a}}_i^* = (1 - c) \cdot \hat{\mathbf{a}}_i + c \cdot f_i(u_\rho) \tag{7}$$

where $\hat{\mathbf{a}}_i$ refers to the i-th column of the estimated mixing matrix $\hat{\mathbf{A}}$ and c is a confidence parameter ranging from 0 to 1. The confidence parameter c in Equation (7) indicates the percentage of weighting of the prior knowledge by means of the expected function $f_i(u_\rho)$. In the limit of $c \to 0$ the original Infomax weight update is used (cf. Equation (6)). It is important to note that for each iteration step only one column in $\hat{\mathbf{A}}$ is updated as expressed in Equation (7) since we do not want to influence the decomposition of the remaining components during the unmixing process. The column in $\hat{\mathbf{A}}$ which entries are most similar to the corresponding expectation function is selected and modified according to Equation (7). As a measure for similarity the kurtosis of the deviation function $d_i = \hat{a}_i - f_i(u_\rho)$ is used:

$$kurt(d_i) = \frac{1}{N} \cdot \sum_{\rho}^{N} \left(\frac{d_{i,\rho} - \bar{d}_i}{\sigma_i} \right)^4 - 3, \tag{8}$$

where $\bar{d}_i$ is the expected value of the deviation function of the i-th component. In the ideal case d_i will be zero (or close to zero); for any deviation at one or more corresponding angles ρ the measure $kurt(d_i)$ will largely be increased. For a subsequent selection of columns in $\hat{\mathbf{A}}$ the column profile with smallest kurtosis value as expressed by Equation (8) is used first. Moreover, if the mean square error (MSE) between the updated column $\hat{a}_i^*$ and the corresponding theoretically expectation function $f_i(u_\rho)$ is less than a predefined tolerance value t the entries of $\hat{a}_i^*$ are fixed. Thus, the MSE is expressed by:

$$MSE(\hat{a}_i^*, f_i(u_\rho)) = \frac{1}{N} \cdot \sum_{\rho}^{N} (\hat{a}_i^*(\rho) - f_i(u_\rho))^2. \tag{9}$$

The basic idea here is that a very small MSE (i.e., $MSE \le t$) in Equation (9) indicates that $\hat{a}_i^*$ and $f_i(u_\rho)$ are very similar, which means that the i-th column in $\hat{\mathbf{A}}$ then represents a source of interest. This approach is repeated for the remaining columns in $\hat{\mathbf{A}}$ until no further components of interest are found. As a stopping criterion for the iteration, a predefined threshold, ε, for the

MSE (with $\varepsilon \gg t$) is used to prevent the algorithm of running into an endless loop. This differentiation of updating $\hat{a}_i^*$ is expressed in Equation (10):

$$\hat{a}_i^* = \begin{cases} (1-c) \cdot \hat{a}_i + c \cdot f_i(u_\rho) & , \; if \; kurt(d_i) < \varepsilon \wedge MSE\left(\hat{a}_i, \; f_i(u_\rho)\right) > t \\ \hat{a}_i & , \; else \end{cases} \tag{10}$$

For the weight update described in Equation (10) the choice of the confidence value c and the tolerance values t and ε should be performed in a representative but independent data set, which is described later.

2.2.1. Evaluation of the signal enhancement

For measuring the noise reduction and signal enhancement in a set of 3D-PLI data after ICA application we use the weighted reduced chi-squared statistic as introduced in [23]. The reduced chi-squared statistic χ^2 involves the variance σ^2 of the observation, where the statistical output is weighted based on the measurement error

$$\chi^2 = \frac{1}{v} \cdot \sum_\rho^N \frac{(I_\rho - f(u_\rho))^2}{\sigma_\rho^2}. \tag{11}$$

Here, I_ρ denote the intensity measured at angle ρ. The variance σ^2 used in Equation (11) was obtained from 100 flat field images, which were independently generated for the image calibration process [22]. The weighted sum over N angles is further normalized by the degrees of freedom v. The normalization ensures a good fit when the reduced chi-square value equals one, which is achieved when the squared difference between the measurement and the expected function resemble the variance of the measurement. In order to measure the signal improvement (and the reduction of noise) through the ICA process the test statistic is determined before $\left(\chi_{raw}^2\right)$ and after $\left(\chi_{ICA}^2\right)$ ICA. Using the ratio of these values and introducing a weight factor ω that penalizes the goodness of fit, whenever a signal component is missing [23]. The weighted test statistic reads as follows:

$$wrGOF(x, y) = \frac{\chi_{raw}^2}{\omega \cdot \chi_{ICA}^2}, \tag{12}$$

with $\omega = \frac{1}{v} \cdot \sum_\rho^N \frac{(f_{raw}(u_\rho) - f_{ICA}(u_\rho))^2}{\sigma_\rho^2} \geq 1$.

The weight factor ω increases when the squared difference between the two expectation functions $f_{raw}(u_\rho)$ and $f_{ICA}(u_\rho)$ (derived from the raw and the ICA filtered PLI data sets, respectively) is large. In case of missed components of interest, the signal strength of the ICA filtered 3D-PLI signal would be largely reduced at corresponding pixel locations. Consequently the expectation function $f_{ICA}(u_p)$ would differ in terms of its amplitude, while the shape of the waveform may be still sinusoidal. The assumption here is that the signal power (across the rotation angles) of the signal of interest is larger compared to noise. The restriction of $\omega \geq 1$ is needed in order to not artificially improve the goodness-of-fit in cases where the two expectation functions $f_{raw}(u_p)$ and $f_{ICA}(u_p)$ are very similar (e.g., at pixel locations with low noise).

2.2.2. Finding the optimal parameters

The optimal parameters c, t and ε for the weight update as described above (cf. Equation (10)), should be determined using a representative but independent data set. In the test data from the same post-mortem brain were used, but from a different microtome section which is not included in the subsequent analysis. The determination of the optimal parameters for cICAP requires the maximization of the weighted goodness-of-fit (wrGOF) values across all pixel locations ($\approx 3.41 \cdot 10^5$ pixels). As a control measure for this requirement the minimal wrGOF value was checked for all trajectories (i.e., the intensity profiles at pixel location x,y) within the brain section. In total we performed 1225 ($=35^2$) cICAP calculations while varying both the confidence value c and the tolerance value t accordingly to the range from 0.0 to 0.7 and 10^{-3} to 10^{-7}, respectively. Figure 3a shows the results of this benchmark run. The largest improvement (cf. blue dot in Figure 3a) was found for the confidence and tolerance values of $c=0.16$ and $t=1.07 \cdot 10^{-6}$, respectively. Once both parameters c and t are fixed the stopping criterion ε, which controls the number of iterations, can be determined. For this task, we investigated the smallest and largest error found in the base functions of $\hat{A}$ by means of the MSE value as expressed by Equation (9). As a reference for the definition of signal components, the user independent component selection tool was used, which is based on the statistically analysis of the base functions as reported in [23]. Throughout all iterations in cICAP the maximal MSE across the columns in matrix $\hat{A}$ that were identified as signal components was found to be well below 0.01. Figure 3b shows that after about 35 iterations the MSE value converges to almost a constant for both the signal (red) and noise components (blue), where both types of components can clearly be identified by means of the corresponding MSE value.

In Figure 4 the progress of changes in the sinusoidal profile of one exemplary basis vector is shown for all 18 iterations (blue) within cICAP. The algorithm converges with a very small fit error (MSE) of $1.07 \cdot 10^{-6}$. The resulting sinusoidal trajectory (black) almost perfectly fits the theoretically expectation function (red).

The process of updating the weight matrix and how a priori knowledge is included in cICAP is shown in Figure 5. Once a basis vector resembles the expectation function under the criteria of $MSE(\hat{a}_i^*) < t$, this basis vector is not changed in further iterations. Note, throughout the optimization the selection of the underlying signal components is automatically included in cICAP and no further user interaction is required.

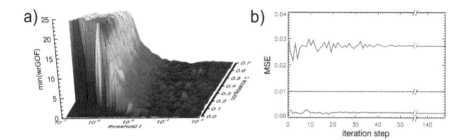

Figure 3. Parameter benchmark run. In (a) the optimal confidence value c and the tolerance value t was determined through a test run of 1225 signal decomposition steps varying both parameters c and t 35 times each through the range from 0.0 to 0.7 and 10^{-3} to 10^{-7}, respectively. As a control measure to find the best parameters, where the goodness-of-fit statistics (wrGOF) is increased at all pixel locations, the largest minimal $wrGOF$ value (blue circle) is determined. The best set of parameters was found for $c=0.16$ and $t=1.07 \cdot 10^{-6}$ with a minimal wrGOF value of about 21. (b) The development of the maximal mean squared error (MSE) is shown for 147 iterations to determine the stopping criterion ε, which controls the number of iterations. The maximal and minimal MSE value is plotted for components reflecting signal of interest (red) and noise components (blue), respectively. After a few iterations the largest MSE value for signal components was found to be well below 1%. Therefore, setting ε to 0.01 both types of components can clearly be identified.

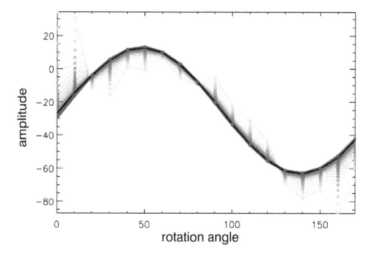

Figure 4. Stepwise changes of one exemplary basis function (changing from light blue to black). After 18 iterations using $cICAP$ the algorithm converges with a very small fit error (MSE) of $1.07 \cdot 10^{-6}$. The resulting sinusoidal trajectory (black) almost perfectly fits the theoretically expectation function (red).

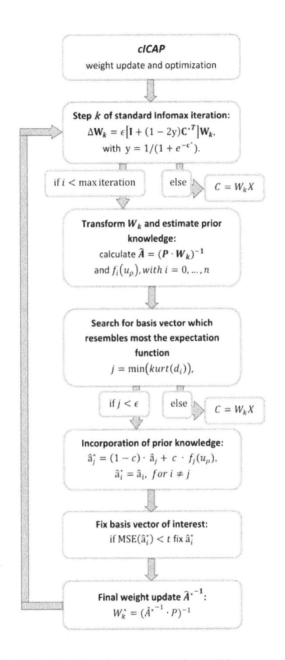

Figure 5. Scheme of the weight matrix update and optimization procedure in *cICAP*.

3. Signal enhancement in 3D-PLI data sets

3.1. Signal acquisition and preprocessing

The performance of *cICAP* was tested on 102 histological sections of one adult human brain acquired from the body donor program of the University of Rostock, Germany, in accordance with legal requirements. The brain was fixed in 4% formalin for 6 months, cryo-protected with glycerin and cut after freezing in a cryostat microtome (Polycut CM 3500, Leica, Germany). The brain was sectioned coronally with slice a thickness of 70 µm. The sections were mounted on glass slides with Aquatex© (Merck, Germany) and cover-slipped. Note that all preparation steps are conforming to preserve the integrity of the birefringent myelin sheaths.

The sections were digitized using the polarimeter setup described in section 1.2. Each brain section was imaged at 18 equidistant rotation angles of the polarimeter covering an angle range between 0° and 170° (Figure 1b). The acquired RGB-colored images have a size of 2776 × 2080 pixels with a pixel size of 64 µm × 64 µm. The intensities were sampled with a dynamic range of 14 bits per color channel. Since the light source of the polarimeter is composed of light-emitting diodes (LED) emitting a narrow-band green wavelength spectrum (central wavelength of 525 nm), only the green channel from the RGB color triplet was used for further analysis.

Before the images were decomposed by ICA, a standardized calibration technique using flat fields was applied, in order to compensate pixel-wise for inhomogeneities across the field of view [22]. In addition, the separation of brain tissue from the non-relevant image background was done by means of the interactive learning and segmentation toolkit (ilastik) [44]. Thus, the following calculations and statistical analyses were solely done on basis of brain tissue measurements.

3.2. Performance on signal decomposition using *cICAP*

To test the performance of the signal decomposition and signal restoration *cICAP* was applied to the data set described in section 3.1. The mean number of pixels used for ICA across the 102 brain sections was found to be $(3.32 \pm 0.95) \cdot 10^5$. The results of signal decomposition and enhancement gained by *cICAP* were compared to the automatic component selection routine, which were recently published in [23], whereas the threshold for this data set was adapted to 2.2.

After the determination of the parameters c, t and ε all values were fixed within *cICAP* and both ICA algorithms were applied to the same set of PLI data for comparison. As shown in Table 1, the identified number of signal components (on average) does not vary dramatically across both algorithms. However, the smallest variability with the fewest number of iterations needed was found in the results of *cICAP*. The number of iterations needed (on average) in *cICAP* was 192, while for the Infomax algorithm using the automatic selection routine it was found to be 406. More importantly, the goodness-of-fit criterion *wrGOF* was found to be largest using *cICAP*. It is important to note that this criterion expresses the signal enhancement (or degradation) after ICA filtering and was calculated for all trajectories (i.e., at each pixel location). If the *wrGOF* value is larger than 1, then noise and artifacts were removed (or suppressed) successfully. In cases, where the signal decomposition fails (or is not optimal) the *wrGOF* value becomes even smaller than 1 (Figure 6). To check the decomposition results for signal degradation after the application of ICA, the minimal *wrGOF* value was calculated. As illustrated in Table 1 a *wrGOF* value smaller than 1 was found in 3.57% and 0.35% of all pixels in the results from Infomax and *cICAP*, respectively.

In general both ICA algorithms produced remarkable decomposition results, where signal enhancement (*wrGOF* ≥ 1) is evident in almost all pixels. However, we found a much better signal decomposition performance in the results of *cICAP*. This is expressed by the fact that the *wrGOF* value was found to be equal or larger than 10 in about 80% of all trajectories, while for the Infomax algorithm it was 39%. For *cICAP* we still found a goodness-of-fit value of larger or equal than 100 in 56% of all pixels. In comparison to the standard Infomax this number drops down to about 15%.

	I) Infomax	II) cICAP
identified ICs (mean)	7.7 ± 4.75	3.8 ± 1.19
number of iterations (mean)	405.5± 32.3	191.8± 23.13
wrGOF (median)	18.8	1910.5
wrGOF < 1 (%)	3.57 %	0.35 %
wrGOF ≥ 10 (%)	38.8 %	80.0 %
wrGOF ≥ 100 (%)	15.1 %	55.6 %

Table 1. Statistical analysis of ICA decomposition results. The signal components for the ICA routine *I* were selected by means of a user independent algorithm (see text).

In Figure 6a pixel locations of a representative section is shown, where the test statistic (*wrGOF*) is larger or equal 300. In this example signal enhancement was evident at all pixel locations (i.e., *wrGOF* > 1; not shown). By focusing on larger values of the test statistic (e.g., *wrGOF* ≥ 300) the figure demonstrates that the enhancement of the optical signals is ensured in particular in the region of the neo-cortex and at the white to gray matter boundary (Figure 6a). This in general is challenging, since in such regions the 3D-PLI signal has low amplitudes and therefore the measured signal has a poor signal-to-noise ratio.

With the introduction of the weighting factor (or penalty factor) as expressed by Equation (12), the test statistic *wrGOF* is sensitive to both, changes in the signal-to-noise ratio as well as in reductions of signal strength after ICA. This in particular will be the case when one or more components of interest are not selected for signal reconstruction (e.g., when the selection is performed manually). As a result, at corresponding pixel locations the *wrGOF* value will be less than 1. The idea behind this is, that the weighted test statistic *wrGOF* accounts for missing gray and white matter components and improvements in SNR, independently to the metric used for identification of components of interest. In Figure 6b such a testing scenario is demonstrated, where one component of interest was manually excluded before the 3D-PLI signal was reconstructed. For this section, 24% of all pixels have a *wrGOF* value below 1.

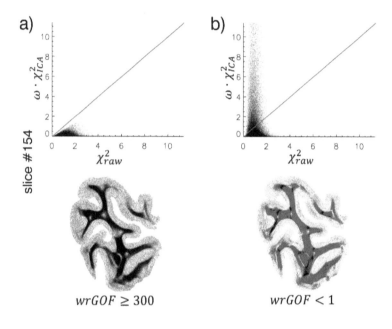

Figure 6. χ^2 ratios and pixel locations illustrating goodness-of-fit values. In a) χ^2 ratios are shown using all components identified by *cICAP*, where the goodness-of-fit statistics was larger than 1 at all pixel locations. In the coronal brain section pixels highlighted in red show locations with goodness-of-fit values larger than 300. b)To demonstrate the effect of being sensitive to missing signal of interest, one identified component was manually deselected. As a result, large areas of white matter structure do show a *wrGOF* value of less than 1 (highlighted in blue).

4. Conclusion

In recent years 3D-polarized light imaging (3D-PLI) has been shown to provide new insights into the organization of the human brain including mapping of the fiber anatomy [15,45,46]. Through advances in the experimental setup of the employed polarimeter, as well as in signal processing, this modality provides unique data sets to explore the 3D fiber architecture in the human brain at a submillimeter resolution [16,47,48]. Though the technique as described here is applicable solely to postmortem brain tissue, the comprehensive description of complex fiber orientations in distinct brain regions (e.g., prevalent fiber crossings) can be used to guide and evaluate fiber tractography algorithms based on diffusion MRI. By this means the fiber orientation maps provided by 3D-PLI might help to optimize the reliability of in-vivo diffusion MRI results. Precise information about the local individual fiber architecture of a patient is of particular interest in case of planning and performing a neurosurgical intervention, for instance.

However, in 3D-PLI the reconstruction of nerve fiber pathways strongly depends on the quality of the measured intensities represented by the so-called light intensity profiles or 3D-PLI signals, respectively. Hence, advanced signal processing tools are required to enable the precise determination of locally prevailing fiber orientations in form of unit vectors defined by the in-section direction angle φ and the out-of-section inclination angle α.

Independent component analysis (ICA) turned out to improve 3D-PLI signals significantly [22,23]. It was shown that ICA is capable of restoring the original birefringent signal by effectively removing noise and artifact components in the measured data. In addition, measures for the qualitative and quantitative evaluation of the 3D-PLI signals before and after the ICA filtering were introduced. In particular, the signal enhancement after ICA based denoising is large at the white to gray matter boundary, where the 3D-PLI signal is weak due to decreasing fiber density when approaching gray matter domains [22].

In *cICAP*, the "constrained ICA for polarized light imaging", the signal decomposition is optimized using a weight update, which incorporates the prior knowledge that the expected signal in 3D-PLI can be modeled utilizing the Jones calculus (cf. Equation (1)). This prior knowledge gives rise to a training of the unmixing procedure in *cICAP*, where the weight matrix update is optimal with respect to the sources of interest (cf. Equation (10)). Utilizing this approach the source separation and identification in *cICAP* is carried out automatically in one routine, where no further component selection tool is needed for subsequent extraction of the signal of interest.

With the introduction of *cICAP* an ICA-based source separation method is available which is optimal for the extraction of the sinusoidal trajectory along different rotation angles in a set of spatially mixed 3D-PLI images. The better quality of the source separation in *cICAP* is reflected by the increased goodness-of-fit statistic (*wrGOF*), which not only takes the improvement in the signal-to-noise ratio (SNR) into account, but also accounts for signal restoration [23].

The dedicated signal processing tool *cICAP* largely contributes to the reliability of 3D-PLI signals and, hence, the accuracy of subsequent fiber tract reconstruction. As a consequence, *cICAP* plays a key role in the 3D-PLI processing chain and helps to establish the so far missing link between the microscopic and the macroscopic characterization of the anatomical connectivity of the human brain.

Acknowledgements

We thank Prof. Dr. A. Wree, Institute for Anatomy, University of Rostock, for providing us with the postmortem human brain.

Author details

Jürgen Dammers[1], Lukas Breuer[1], Giuseppe Tabbì[2] and Markus Axer[2]

1 Institute of Neuroscience and Medicine, Medical Imaging Physics, INM-4, Forschungszentrum Jülich, Jülich, Germany

2 Institute of Neuroscience and Medicine, Structural and Functional Organisation of the Brain, INM-1, Forschungszentrum Jülich, Jülich, Germany

References

[1] Mesulam, M. Foreword. In: Schmahmann JD, Pandya DN, editors. Fiber pathways of the brain. Oxford University Press; (2006).

[2] Kötter, R. Handbook of brain connectivity. In: Jirsa VK, McIntosh AR, editors. Berlin New York: Springer; (2007). page , 149-1167.

[3] Sporns, O, Tononi, G, & Kötter, R. The human connectome: A structural description of the human brain. PLoS computational biology. Public Library of Science; (2005). Sep;, 1(4), 245-51.

[4] Johansen-berg, H. Behrens TEJ. Diffusion MRI: From Quantitative Measurement to In-vivo Neuroanatomy. Academic Press; (2009). page 490.

[5] Jones, D. K. Diffusion MRI: Theory, Methods, and Applications. Jones DK, editor. Oxford University Press; (2011). page 624.

[6] Türe, U, Yasargil, M. G, Friedman, A. H, & Al-mefty, O. Fiber dissection technique: lateral aspect of the brain. Neurosurgery. (2000). Aug;, 47(2), 417-27.

[7] Klingler, J. Erleichterung der makroskopischen Präparation des Gehirns durch den Gefrierprozess. Schweizer Archiv für Neurologie und Psychiatrie. (1935).

[8] Bürgel, U, Amunts, K, Hoemke, L, Mohlberg, H, Gilsbach, J. M, & Zilles, K. White matter fiber tracts of the human brain: three-dimensional mapping at microscopic resolution, topography and intersubject variability. NeuroImage. Department of Neurosurgery, RWTH Aachen University, D-52074 Aachen, Germany.; (2006). Feb 15;, 29(4), 1092-105.

[9] Flechsig, P. Developmental (myelongenetic) localisation of the cerebral cortex in the human subject. Lancet. (1901).

[10] Fink, R. P, & Heimer, L. Two methods for selective silver impregnation of degenerating axons and their synaptic endings in the central nervous system. Brain Research. (1967). Apr;, 4(4), 369-74.

[11] Clarke, S, & Miklossy, J. Occipital cortex in man: organization of callosal connections, related myelo- and cytoarchitecture, and putative boundaries of functional visual areas. J. Comp. Neurol. (1990).

[12] Burkhalter, A, Bernardo, K. L, & Charles, V. Development of local circuits in human visual cortex. The Journal of neuroscience- the official journal of the Society for Neuroscience. (1993). May;, 13(5), 1916-31.

[13] Lanciego, J, & Wouterlood, F. Neuroanatomical tract-tracing methods beyond 2000: what's now and next. Journal of Neuroscience Methods. (2000). Nov;, 103(1), 1-2.

[14] Schmahmann, J, & Pandya, D. Fiber Pathways of the Brain. Oxford University Press; (2010). page 672.

[15] Axer, M, Grässel, D, Kleiner, M, Dammers, J, Dickscheid, T, Reckfort, J, et al. High-resolution fiber tract reconstruction in the human brain by means of three-dimensional polarized light imaging. Frontiers in neuroinformatics. (2011). Jan;, 5(34), 1-13.

[16] Axer, M, Amunts, K, Grässel, D, Palm, C, Dammers, J, Axer, H, et al. A novel approach to the human connectome: ultra-high resolution mapping of fiber tracts in the brain. NeuroImage. (2011). Jan;, 54(2), 1091-101.

[17] Axer, H, Beck, S, Axer, M, Schuchardt, F, Heepe, J, Flücken, A, et al. Microstructural analysis of human white matter architecture using polarized light imaging: views from neuroanatomy. Frontiers in neuroinformatics. (2011). Jan;, 5(28), 1-12.

[18] Schmitt, F. O, & Bear, R. S. The optical properties of vertebrate nerve axons as related to fiber size. Journal of Cellular and Comparative Physiology. (1937). Feb;, 9(2), 261-73.

[19] Schmidt, W. J. Zur Doppelbrechung des Nervenmarks. Zeitschrift für wissenschaftliche Mikroskopie. (1923). , 41, 29-38.

[20] Göthlin, G. F. Die doppelbrechenden Eigenschaften des Nervengewebes. Kungliga Svenska Vetenskapsakademiens. (1913). Handlingar(51).

[21] Jones, R. C. A New Calculus for the Treatment of Optical Systems. Journal of the Optical Society of America. (1941). Jul;, 31(7), 500-3.

[22] Dammers, J, Axer, M, Grässel, D, Palm, C, Zilles, K, Amunts, K, et al. Signal enhancement in polarized light imaging by means of independent component analysis. NeuroImage. (2010). Jan;, 49(2), 1241-8.

[23] Dammers, J, Breuer, L, Axer, M, Kleiner, M, Eiben, B, Grässel, D, et al. Automatic identification of gray and white matter components in polarized light imaging. NeuroImage. (2012). Jan 16;, 59(2), 1338-47.

[24] Beckmann, C. F, & Smith, S. M. Probabilistic independent component analysis for functional magnetic resonance imaging. IEEE Transactions on Medical Imaging. (2004). Feb;, 23(2), 137-52.

[25] Cong, F, Kalyakin, I, Ahuttunen-scott, T, Li, H, Lyytinen, H, & Ristaniemi, T. Single-trial based Independent Component Analysis on Mismatch Negativity in Children. International Journal of Neural Systems. (2010).

[26] Esposito, F, Formisano, E, Seifritz, E, Goebel, R, Morrone, R, Tedeschi, G, et al. Spatial independent component analysis of functional MRI time-series: to what extent do results depend on the algorithm used? Human brain mapping. (2002). Jul;, 16(3), 146-57.

[27] Hild, K. E, & Nagarajan, S. S. Source localization of EEG/MEG data by correlating columns of ICA and lead field matrices. IEEE transactions on bio-medical engineering. (2009). Nov;, 56(11), 2619-26.

[28] Bartlett, M. S. Information maximization in face processing. Neurocomputing. (2007). Aug;70(13-15):2204-17.

[29] Dammers, J, Schiek, M, Boers, F, Silex, C, Zvyagintsev, M, Pietrzyk, U, et al. Integration of amplitude and phase statistics for complete artifact removal in independent components of neuromagnetic recordings. IEEE Trans. Biomed. Eng. (2008). Oct;, 55(10), 2353-62.

[30] Escudero, J, Hornero, R, Abásolo, D, & Fernández, A. Quantitative evaluation of artifact removal in real magnetoencephalogram signals with blind source separation. Annals of biomedical engineering. Springer Netherlands; (2011). Aug 21;, 39(8), 2274-86.

[31] Li, Y, Ma, Z, Lu, W, & Li, Y. Automatic removal of the eye blink artifact from EEG using an ICA-based template matching approach. Physiological measurement. (2006). Apr;, 27(4), 425-36.

[32] Mantini, D, Franciotti, R, Romani, G. L, & Pizzella, V. Improving MEG source localizations: an automated method for complete artifact removal based on independent component analysis. NeuroImage. (2008). Mar;, 40(1), 160-73.

[33] Nikulin, V V, Nolte, G, & Curio, G. A novel method for reliable and fast extraction of neuronal EEG/MEG oscillations on the basis of spatio-spectral decomposition. NeuroImage. (2011). Apr 15;, 55(4), 1528-35.

[34] Huang, D-S, & Mi, J-X. A New Constrained Independent Component Analysis Method. IEEE Transactions on Neural Networks. (2007). Sep;, 18(5), 1532-5.

[35] Hesse, C. W. On estimating the signal subspace dimension of high-density multi-channel magnetoencephalogram measurements. Conference proceedings©: Annual International Conference of the IEEE Engineering in Medicine and Biology Society. IEEE Engineering in Medicine and Biology Society. Lyon, France. (2007). Jan;, 6228-31.

[36] Liu, J, Ghassemi, M. M, Michael, A. M, Boutte, D, Wells, W, Perrone-bizzozero, N, et al. An ICA with reference approach in identification of genetic variation and associated brain networks. Frontiers in human neuroscience. (2012). Jan;, 6(21), 1-10.

[37] Barriga, E. S, Pattichis, M, Ts, o D, Abramoff, M, Kardon, R, Kwon, Y, et al. Independent component analysis using prior information for signal detection in a functional imaging system of the retina. Medical image analysis. (2011). Feb;, 15(1), 35-44.

[38] Hesse, C. W, & James, C. J. On semi-blind source separation using spatial constraints with applications in EEG analysis. IEEE transactions on bio-medical engineering. (2006). Dec;53(12 Pt 1):2525-34.

[39] Stone, J V. Independent Component Analysis: A Tutorial Introduction. MIT Press; (2004). page 211.

[40] Hyvärinen, A, Karhunen, J, & Oja, E. Independent component analysis. John Wiley and Sons; (2001). page 481.

[41] Bell, A. J. Sejnowski T errence J. An information-maximization approach to blind separation and blind deconvolution. Neural computation. MIT Press; (1995). Nov;, 7(6), 1129-59.

[42] Brown, G. D, Yamada, S, & Sejnowski, T. J. Independent component analysis at the neural cocktail party. Trends in neurosciences. (2001). Jan;, 24(1), 54-63.

[43] Amari, S, Cichocki, A, & Yang, H. H. A new learning algorithm for blind signal separation. In: Tourezky D, Mozer M, Hazzelmo M, editors. Advances in neural information processing systems. (1996). page , 757-763.

[44] Sommer, C, Straehle, C, Kothe, U, & Hamprecht, F. A. Ilastik: Interactive learning and segmentation toolkit. 2011 IEEE International Symposium on Biomedical Imaging: From Nano to Macro. IEEE; (2011). page , 230-3.

[45] Axer, H, Klingner, C. M, & Prescher, A. Fiber anatomy of dorsal and ventral language streams. Brain and language. (2012). May 23;

[46] Larsen, L, Griffin, L. D, Grässel, D, Witte, O. W, & Axer, H. Polarized light imaging of white matter architecture. Microscopy Research and Technique. (2007). Oct;, 70(10), 851-63.

[47] Gräßel DAxer M, Palm C, Dammers J, Amunts K, Pietrzyk U, et al. Visualization of Fiber Tracts in the Postmortem Human Brain by Means of Polarized Light. Neuro-Image. (2009). Jul;47(Supplement 1):142.

[48] Palm C Axer M Gräßel D, Dammers J, Lindemeyer J, Zilles K, et al. Towards Ultra-High Resolution Fibre Tract Mapping of the Human Brain- Registration of Polarised Light Images and Reorientation of Fibre Vectors. Frontiers in human neuroscience. FRONTIERS RES FOUND; (2010). Jan;, 4(9), 1-16.

Chapter 5

Neuroimaging of Epilepsy: EEG-fMRI in the Presurgical Evaluation of Focal Epilepsy

Mirko Avesani, Silvia Giacopuzzi and
Antonio Fiaschi

Additional information is available at the end of the chapter

1. Introduction

Epilepsies of surgical interest are focal and drug-resistant forms associated with various different conditions (malformations, stroke, tumors, infectious and/or inflammatory processes, brain injuries). There is mounting evidence that early resective surgery can achieve seizure-free status or reduce seizure frequency. The main challenge in the presurgical assessment of patients with epilepsy is to localize the area of seizure onset (the epileptogenic zone) and to distinguish it from lesional and interictal foci (the irritative zone) because it is only by treating the epileptogenic zone that seizure freedom or a reduction in events may be attained (Thorton, 2010).

This is explained by the fact that since the interictal focus is larger than the epileptogenic zone, the epileptogenic zone does not always overlap the lesional area and the epileptogenic focus is often larger than lesional area (Avesani, 2008/a; Manganotti, 2008; Thorton, 2010). In general, interictal epileptic discharges may affect brain areas well beyond the presumed region in which they are generated (Gotman, 2008). While resection of the lesional area alone is not sufficient, neither can the entire interictal focus be removed due to the high risk of cognitive, motor, sensitive or language deficits.

Presurgical evaluation involves invasive investigation by stereoelectroencephalography (SEEG) performed after other routine exams (standard EEG, video-EEG, functional neuroimaging) to identify the interictal focus within the epileptogenic zone. The lesional area, instead, is nowadays studied with advanced MRI techniques developed to better identify the interictal focus.

2. Functional imaging in epilepsy

Functional imaging refers to noninvasive methods to identify the interictal focus and the epileptogenic zone which, in a subsequent step, is studied with an invasive technique (SEEG, electrocortical mapping). The most widely used are:

- positron-emission tomography (PET)

- single-photon-emission computed tomography (SPECT)

- magnetic resonance spectroscopy (MRS)

- functional magnetic imaging (fMRI)

These techniques allow the study of a specific area of the brain, obviating the need for invasive studies of the entire brain. PET and SPECT were initially utilized for this purpose. While both provide a better knowledge of the brain's functional anatomy, they rarely allow for a precise localization of an epileptogenic focus, making them less useful for surgical planning (Marks, 1992; Henry, 1993; Newton, 1995).

The rationale for SPECT is based on its ability to reveal, in vivo, the volume distribution of a radiotracer after intravenous injection, and to evaluate, quantitatively and qualitatively, regional brain perfusion (Devous, 2005). The application of SPECT in epilepsy derives from a known association between an electrical event and brain perfusion: brain perfusion increases during the ictal phase and decreases during the interictal phase. Studies using dynamic and static SPECT have demonstrated interictal temporal hypoperfusion in 50% patients with temporal-lobe epilepsy (TLE). Nevertheless, the limitation of this technique is that 5-10% of patients demonstrate contralateral hypoperfusion, which raises the risk of false localization (Krausz, 1991). The localization power of SPECT during the interictal phase is, therefore, variable, with a sensitivity of 36% and a specificity of 95% (Engel, 1982). For this reason, SPECT is useful as a comparative study of ictal and interictal perfusion in selected patients. When applied during a seizure, it demonstrates the dynamic aspect of the seizure during its development. Unlike interictal studies, ictal SPECT, in both temporal and extratemporal epilepsy, is accurate in localizing an epileptogenic focus. During the ictal phase it can reveal, with a sensitivity of 70-95%, hyperperfusion in an area activated by seizures (Engel, 1983; Lee, 1994).

PET is a powerful imaging technique to quantify, in vivo and noninvasively, cerebral blood flow, metabolism and receptorial links. Its main application derives from the need to identify epileptogenic foci in patients with drug-resistant epilepsy, potential candidates for surgical treatment to control or abolish drug-resistant focal seizures. In up to 20-30% of such patients, who are candidates for surgical treatment, the MRI exam is negative (Duncan, 1997) because microscopic structural malformations, identifiable only by histological study, are not detectable with conventional MRI (Kuzniecky, 1991). Using [11C]flumazenil positron-emission tomography ([11C]FMZ-PET), Hammers studied 18 patients with TLE and normal MRI: 16 demonstrated abnormalities in the binding of [11] C-FMZ in the temporal lobe; 7 of these were concordant with clinical and standard EEG data; 3 patients underwent surgical treatment of the anterior temporal lobe, with marked clinical improvement. The neuropathological data revealed microdysgenesis not detected by MRI (Hammers, 2002).

In patients with focal seizures, glucose metabolism and cerebral blood flow in a particular focal region are increased during an ictal event (Engel, 1983). In the postictal phase, hyperperfusion gradually returns to the basal level, but glucose metabolism remains elevated for 24-48 hours after seizure termination (Leiderman, 1994). In the interictal phase, PET demonstrates a decrease in glucose metabolism and cerebral blood flow in the epileptogenic focus. Studies using 18-fluoro-2-deoxy-glucose-positron emission tomography (18F-FDG-PET) demonstrated hypometabolism in the temporal lobe in 60-90% of patients with interictal spikes (Duncan, 1997). Nevertheless, an area with abnormal cerebral blood flow and metabolism, as detected with PET, is larger than the real structural anomaly generating an epileptogenic focus probably because of deafferentation phenomena in the surrounding neurons in areas of seizure propagation (Duncan, 1997). Since this carries the risk of false localization, PET is regarded as being more suitable for studying lateralization than localization (Tai, 2004).

MR spectroscopy can be utilized in the noninvasive assessment of specific cerebral metabolites. In epilepsy the aim is to determine a focal change in the main metabolites deriving from focal brain dysfunction. The initial aim of the method was to delimit the epileptogenic focus and to analyze the distant repercussions of the lesion and the focus. For example, spectroscopy can reveal bilateral hippocampal abnormalities in unilateral mesial temporal sclerosis (MTS). The technique has demonstrated its utility in identifying metabolic dysfunction in patients with TLE. Nevertheless, owing to its high sensitivity, metabolic abnormalities may be revealed in regions without an epileptogenic focus, making it difficult to distinguish the causal abnormalities from their consequences (Ruben, 2005).

In patients with drug-resistant TLE, spectroscopy demonstrated a lower N-acetyl aspartate/ creatine (NAA/Cr) ratio, a reliable marker of neuronal integrity, in the ipsi- and contralateral lobes, and this finding correlated negatively with seizure duration (Bernasconi, 2002). Patients with frequent generalized seizures were noted to have a lower NAA/Cr ratio than those with rare or no seizures. Another interesting finding was the demonstration of reversible dysfunction in the cortical area after surgical treatment (Hugg, 1996). What all this suggests is that seizures may induce additional neuronal damage that will progress with the duration of epilepsy. From this point of view, spectroscopy may be useful as a metabolic marker of disease progression. In the future, it may be possible to decide whether evidence of disease progression on spectroscopy may be sufficient to suggest a change of therapy (Petroff, 2002).

Functional MRI (fMRI) provides high-resolution images using the classical principles of MRI, with the difference that signal recording exploits the paramagnetic properties of hemoglobin when its iron atom changes from Fe^{3+} (oxygenated hemoglobin) to Fe^{2+} (deoxygenated hemoglobin). Only Fe^{2+} has the ability to locally modify the magnetic state of cerebral tissues (Berns, 1999). Activation of a cerebral area causes both oxidative metabolism and local cerebral blood flow to increase, leading to greater oxygen extraction by the tissues. This results in a local increase of deoxyhemoglobin. Functional MRI reveals the activation of a cerebral area from the higher level of deoxyhemoglobin compared to the basal condition. And it does this indirectly by measuring the vascular response to activation of the cerebral area under study.

The response has a variable latency (from 3-5 to 10 seconds), which is why this kind of information is defined as "functional", and the recorded signal, related to hemoglobin oxygenation, is defined as BOLD (Blood Oxygen Level Dependent) (Ogawa, 1990; Prichard, 1994).

fMRI works by comparing the images obtained in rest condition with those acquired during a task. Whether and to what extent physiological correlates match different BOLD phases (Menon, 2001) continues to fuel debate, though studies suggest that the fMRI signal is closely related to neuronal activation (Logothetis, 2001). The method was first applied to localize areas associated with motor, sensory and cognitive functions in epileptic patients and to obtain a precise localization of these functions in the presurgical evaluation of epilepsy (Puce, 1995; Binder, 1996; Dupon, 2002).

3. EEG-fMRI

This noninvasive technique provides reliable information to localize cerebral regions generating interictal epileptic activity. It involves the simultaneous recording of EEG and fMRI. With ongoing refinement of the technology (first of all removal of magnetic field artifact on EEG), initial technical limitations have been overcome (Ives, 1993). EEG-fMRI permits the study cerebral activation and deactivation related to infra-clinical spikes by comparing EEG with spiked activity against EEG without abnormalities (Krakow, 1999 and 2001; Lazeyras 2000; Archer, 2003).

Research to date has investigated lesional epilepsy in the temporal region in particular, the most frequent cause of epilepsy of surgical interest. Up until several years ago, triggered EEG-fMRI was used. EEG was recorded during a scanning session, and fMRI acquisition was performed when a neurologist identified, on line, interictal (spikes, polyspikes, spike waves) activity on EEG. Acquisition was performed after a fixed latency (3-5 seconds) from detected interictal activity, which was decided before starting acquisition. The technique had several limitations: it was based on the concept of standardized cerebral hemodynamic activity, even if we know that such activity varies widely (from 3 up to 10 seconds); analysis had to be performed offline using, as a task, spikes with different morphology; and the temporal dynamics of hemodynamic responses could not be identified. Owing to these limitations, early studies with triggered EEG-fMRI (Krakow, 1999 and 2001) showed low sensitivity (60%) in detecting hemodynamic activation related to interictal activity.

Later studies (Lazeyras, 2001; Lemieux, 2001; Al-Asmi, 2003) demonstrated the superiority of continuous EEG-fMRI based on offline analysis after simultaneous EEG recording during a fMRI scanning session and following artifact removal. This development brought about clear advantages: since it was no longer necessary to decide beforehand which abnormal events were to be studied (and recorded) during a single acquisition, the temporal evolution of activations (after 1 to 10 seconds) could be identified and pathophysiological hypotheses about their propagation postulated. Continuous EEG-fMRI detects activation with a sensitivity of 80%.

Numerous studies have applied continuous EEG-fMRI to investigate various different epileptic syndromes (Boor, 2003; Salek-Haddadi, 2003 and 2006; Bagshaw, 2004 and 2006; Aghakhani, 2004 and 2005; Gotman, 2004 and 2005; Kobayashi, 2005 and 2006; Laufs, 2006; Di Bonaventura, 2006; Vaudano, 2009). Some studied focal epilepsies, while others examined idiopathic generalized forms underlying absence seizures.

4. EEG-fMRI in absence seizures

The application of EEG-fMRI in idiopathic generalized epilepsy (IGE), for evident technical problems, is limited to absence seizures or nonconvulsive status, to analyze the network underlying impaired consciousness related to generalized spike wave (GSW) discharges. Clinically, absences are characterized by a blank stare and impaired consciousness. Activities requiring vigilant attention have been coupled with a lesser likelihood of absences, whereas an increased frequency of seizures during relaxation is well established (Andermann, 2000; Guey, 1969). These findings suggest a causal link between changes in the level of awareness and the occurrence of GSW discharges.

Recent functional imaging studies have revealed the existence of a set of brain regions which show increased functional and metabolic activity during rest, compared to attention-demanding tasks (Raichle, 2000; Mazoyer, 2001). Involved brain areas (the posterior cingulated cortex, the precuneus, the medial prefrontal cortex, the mid-dorsolateral prefrontal and the anterior temporal cortices) have been hypothesized to constitute the so-called default mode network (DMN) (Raichle, 2000). Decreased DMN activity during cognitive tasks indicates that the network sustains spontaneous thought processes or self-oriented mental activity that characterizes the brain's resting state.

Additionally, the precuneus/posterior cingulate node has been recently demonstrated to have the highest degree of interactions (as shown by a partial correlation approach to fMRI data) with the rest of the DMN (Frasson, 2008), suggesting a pivotal role of this area within the network. This interpretation is in line with evidence from previous PET studies that this brain region, and the precuneus in particular, has the highest metabolic rate, consuming 35% more glucose than any other area of the cerebral cortex at rest (Gusnard, 2001).

The DMN shows decreased activity during both attention-demanding tasks and states of reduced vigilance and, especially in the posteromedial cortical regions, during altered states of consciousness (Laureys, 2004; Faymonville, 2006). From these observations, several authors (Cavanna, 2006 and 2007; Boly, 2008) suggested a pivotal role of the posteromedial cortical region in self-consciousness inside the DMN.

EEG-correlated functional magnetic resonance imaging (EEG-fMRI) studies have shown a common pattern of BOLD signal decrease in the precuneus and other DMN areas, together with an increase in the thalamic BOLD signal, during ictal and interictal GSW discharges (Aghakhani, 2004; Archer, 2003; Gotman, 2005; Hamandi, 2006; Laufs, 2006; Salek-Haddadi, 2003; De Tiège, 2007; Labate, 2005). Decreased cerebral blood flow consistent with a decrease in neuronal activity was demonstrated in DMN regions during GSW discharges (Hamandi, 2008). Therefore, these relative BOLD signal decreases can be interpreted as a transitory suspension of the brain's "default state" which occurs in association with an altered level of awareness observed during GSW discharges and absences, respectively (Gotman, 2005; Hamandi, 2006; Laufs, 2006; Salek-Haddadi, 2003).

The pathophysiological substrate of GSW remains enigmatic. Studies in animals and humans have tried to answer persistent questions about the putative role of the thalamus and cortex as generators. Data from invasive recordings and manipulations in well-validated genetic models of absence epilepsy have lent support to the hypothesis that absence seizures are of cortical origin (Steriade, 1998; Meeren, 2002 and 2005; Polack, 2007; Holmes, 2004; Tucker, 2007).

Following on the suggestion of the involvement of dorsal cortical regions (particularly the posterior-medial cortical regions) in GSW discharges from neuroimaging studies (Gotman, 2005; Hamandi, 2006; Laufs, 2006; Salek-Haddadi, 2003) and their role in conscious awareness (Faymonville, 2006; Boly, 2008), a recent work (Vaudano, 2009) attempted to elucidate the interaction between these areas and the (frontal)cortical-thalamic loop by means of dynamic causal modeling (DCM) to study effective connectivity based on simultaneously recorded EEG-fMRI data in 7 patients with GSW discharges.

The results of this study are consistent with the concept of the precuneus as a key region that changes its activity with altered states of vigilance, thus influencing the occurrence of gener-alized seizures: changes in the precuneus state (an increase or decrease in its neuronal activity), which reflects spontaneous fluctuations in awareness, act on the thalamic-(frontal) cortical network, facilitating the development of GSW. This contrasts with previous observations (Gotman, 2005; Hamandi, 2006; Laufs, 2006) that decreases in precuneal activity reflect the semiology of impaired consciousness and are a consequence of GSW.

A similar hypothesis was advanced by Archer et al. (Archer, 2003) who observed a significant posterior cingulate negative BOLD response in 5 IGE patients with interictal GSW discharges but no BOLD signal changes in the thalamus or prefrontal cortex. The authors suggested that decreases in posterior cingulate activity and associated regions may be involved in the initiation of GSW activity.

Additionally, a fMRI study showed a BOLD signal decrease in the posterior cingulate in IGE subjects following photic stimulation whether or not GSW activity occurred, while the control subjects showed no change in this region (Hill, 1999). Such changes would be consistent with a decrease in posterior cingulate activity being a precursor (or facilitator) of GSW activity rather than a secondary phenomenon. The posterior cingulate cortex is adjacent to the precuneus and some authors would define it as part of the precuneal cortical area (Frackowiak, 1997; Frasson, 2008).

Current thinking about the pathophysiology of GSW has it that the neuronal state of the precuneus, and the level of awareness, may reflect a "physiological initiator" of generalized synchronous discharges. In this connection, EEG-fMRI adds electrophysiological data to GSW generation and precuneal involvement where, besides the scant evidence for a strict conse-quentiality between a particular state of vigilance and the occurrence of GSW discharges, there is a notable lack of studies on the possible role of cortical structures (particularly the precuneus) other than the thalamus and frontal cortex in GSW.

Unlike surface electrophysiological recordings, fMRI studies with concurrent EEG in patients with GSW discharges have shown common hemodynamic changes not only in the thalamus and frontal cortex, but also in the precuneus and other brain regions (including the fronto-parietal association cortices) of the DMN (Aghakhani, 2004; Archer, 2003; Gotman, 2005; Laufs, 2007). Moreover, fMRI's relatively homogeneous sensitivity across the brain compared to that of scalp EEG may explain why recent EEG-fMRI studies have been able to reveal precuneal involvement in epilepsies characterized by impaired consciousness and associated with GSW (Gotman, 2005; Hamandi, 2006; Laufs, 2006).

In brief, there is an active role in generalized epilepsy for the precuneus, a region previously neglected in electrophysiological studies of GSW. DCM based on EEG-fMRI data has shown that the precuneus is not only strongly connected with the frontal cortex and the thalamus but also that the neuronal activity in this area may facilitate epileptic activity within a thalamo-cortical loop, the existence of which is well established. These findings suggest that GSW may arise through the direct influence of the neuronal state of the precuneus associated with spontaneous changes in the level of awareness.

5. EEG-fMRI in focal seizures: Introduction

5.1. Interictal focal spiked activity correlated BOLD signal changes: Aims and results

EEG-fMRI provides insight into the pathophysiology of changes in the level of awareness during GSW discharges in absence seizures; however, the practical usefulness of technique resides in the study of focal epilepsy, especially if drug resistant and associated with a condition which, if amenable to removal, could achieve seizure freedom or a reduction of frequency. Numerous studies have applied EEG-fMRI to focal seizures to identify the interictal focus and the ictal onset zone (Krakow 1999 and 2001; Boor, 2003; Salek Haddadi, 2006; Bagshaw, 2004 and 2006; Aghakani, 2005; Kobayashi, 2005 and 2006). Some also applied SEEG and electrocortical mapping to study areas previously identified with EEG-fMRI and confirmed co-localization between interictal events (IEDs) and hemodynamic activation detected on fMRI (Krakow, 1999; Kobayashi, 2006; Benar, 2006).

All these studies analyzed patients with spiked activity on focal EEG (spikes, spikes and waves, polyspikes) that differed in frequency. It was then suggested that a limiting factor to obtain sufficient BOLD activation is IED frequency. Two studies (Krakow, 1999 and 2001) proposed 1 IED/minute as the minimum value to obtain sufficient activation. But because a lower frequency does not have sufficient power to stimulate an IED-correlated BOLD signal change, the sensitivity of the technique is very low. More recent studies applied EEG-fMRI to compare the location of IED-correlated BOLD signal change with the resected area and postoperative outcome (Thorton, 2010). Seven out of 10 surgically treated patients were seizure-free following surgery and the area of maximal BOLD signal change was concordant with resection in 6 out of 7 patients. In the remaining 3 patients with reduced seizure frequency post-surgically, the areas of significant IED-correlated BOLD signal change lay outside the resection, thus confirming that the epileptogenic zone (to be removed) is different from the lesional area.

5.2. Interictal focal slow wave activity correlated BOLD changes: The first case reports

Although some studies analyzed focal epilepsies (Liu, 2008), focal slow-wave activity as a marker of activation of cerebral blood flow was initially studied in only two single case reports (Laufs, 2006/a; Avesani 2008/a-b). The one additionally used SEEG to demonstrate co-localization between IEDs and fMRI activation. The second, our case report (Avesani 2008/a), involved a patient with temporal lobe epilepsy (TLE) due to a cavernoma, who had undergone surgical treatment without attaining freedom of seizures. This woman had no medical history of note until the age of 24 years (1975), when symptoms characterized by painful sensations including a lightening stabbing pain developed in the left parietal region of the head, preceded by absence attacks lasting 30 seconds. After seizures she always experienced profound weakness. Her seizures recurred at a variable rate, ranging from more than one a day to one every 10-15 days. During the seizure-free periods she remained healthy. The EEG at that time was negative for an interictal focus. In 1986, when the patient was 35 years old, the EEG disclosed an interictal focus in left temporal regions, characterized by very frequent, and polymorphous, theta-delta activity in association with sharp waves, blocked by eye opening and without contralateral diffusion. Subsequent EEG confirmed the irritative focus in the left fronto-temporal region. When the patient was 37-year-old she began therapy with phenobar-bitone (PB) and carbamazepine (CBZ), benefiting from a decrease in seizure intensity (but not frequency). A computed tomographic (CT) brain scan disclosed a mild, non-homogeneous, subcortical hyperdensity on the mesial side of the left temporal lobe, containing rough calcifications with no contrast enhancement. An MRI scan revealed two small lesions in the left temporal lobe, similar to cavernomas (one anterior, in the Sylvian fissure and another posterior, in the paratrigonal region). The patient underwent surgery but the partial seizures remained unchanged. Treatment with PB and CBZ was therefore continued. Twelve years later (2002), another MRI scan revealed three small independent cavernomas in the left temporal lobe (left temporo-basal, left temporo-mesial, and in the left post-central gyrus). A year later (2003), bleeding of the large lesion (localized in the left temporo-basal region) caused the patient to be re-admitted to the neurosurgical ward to undergo a second operation. Despite repeat surgery the seizures continued so she needed further therapy. A following MRI scan (2005), confirmed the presence of the previous cavernomas without bleeding.

Using interictal focus of slow waves recorded in the left temporal region as a trigger of activation (Fig. 1), we obtained activation in the left posterior cortical region around the poro-encephalic cavity (residual of previous surgical treatment) (Fig. 2). Our findings confirmed observations by Thorton of 3 patients in whom surgical treatment failed to achieve seizure freedom: in these situations areas of significant IED correlated BOLD signal change lay outside the resection (Thorton, 2010).

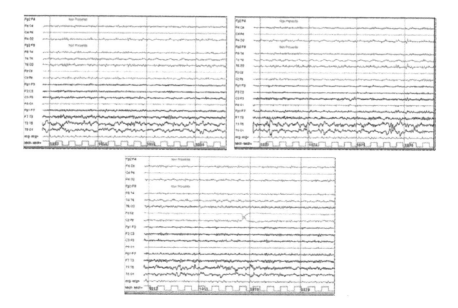

Figure 1. Interictal EEG of patient affected by cavernosa. Focal IEDs in left temporal region

6. EEG fMRI in focal seizures: The first study of interictal slow wave activity correlated bold changes

6.1. Patients enrolled in the study

In a previous study involving 8 patients with focal slow-wave interictal discharges on EEG (Manganotti, 2008), we suggested that an IED-correlated BOLD change triggered by interictal slow-wave activity could be obtained if the focal activity is frequent (about 2 IEDs/min). The study was primarily designed to verify whether the interictal slow waves originating from an EEG interictal focus were sufficient to increase cerebral blood flow in a spatially related brain area. To do so, using EEG-fMRI, we investigated BOLD responses to IEDs characterized by focal interictal slow-wave activity in patients with partial epilepsy.

We also wanted to understand whether, in patients with lesional epilepsy, fMRI-BOLD activation areas were correlated with lesions previously identified with standard MRI. We then investigated whether EEG-fMRI could document the spatial relationship between the interictal zone and the ictal onset zone in patients with interictal focal slow-wave discharges arising from a known epileptogenic lesion (i.e., the lesional area).

To obtain a homogeneous study sample, 8 patients with focal epilepsy were selected from among patients hospitalized in our epilepsy ward whose routine EEG recordings showed frequent focal IEDs manifesting as 5-6 Hz focal EEG activity (slow waves, slow spike waves, high-amplitude slow waves), over a few lateralized electrodes. Three of the 8 patients selected

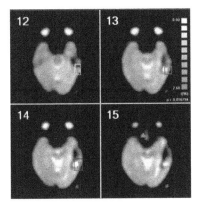

Results of data analysis in 2D reconstruction

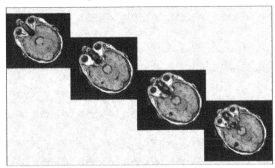

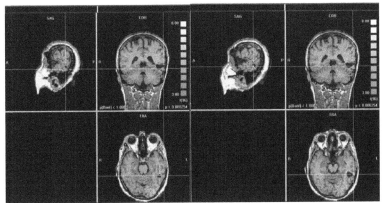

Results of data analysis in 3D recontruction

Figure 2. Interitcal focal slow wave activity correlated BOLD activation in patient affected by cavernoma: results of data analysis both in 2D and in 3D recontruction

for study had a structural lesion on MRI: 2 patients with hippocampal atrophy secondary to mesial temporal sclerosis (MTS) and 1 patient with a cavernous angioma. Among the remaining 5 patients, 1 patient had cryptogenic epilepsy and 4 patients had nonlesional (idiopathic) epilepsy. Routine EEG showed slow-wave activity in 1 patient with MTS (P4), the patient with cryptogenic epilepsy (P2) and the one with idiopathic epilepsy (P7); slow spike waves were observed in the patient with a cavernoma (P3) and the 2 patients with idiopathic epilepsy (P5 and P8); high-amplitude slow-waves (> 130 µV) were noted in 1 patient with idiopathic epilepsy (P6) and the second patient with MTS (P1) (Table 1).

Patients	Type of Epilepsy	Standard MRI findings	IED morphology	Irritative focus
1	Lesional	MTS	HASW	T3-T5
2	Cryptogenic	Negative	SW	T3-T5
3	Lesional	Cavernoma	SPSW	T5
4	Lesional	MTS	SW	T4-T6
5	Idiopathic	Negative	SPSW	O1
6	Idiopathic	Negative	HASW	T4-T6
7	Idiopathic	Negative	SW	F7
8	Idiopathic	Negative	HASPSW	T4-T6

MTS denotes mesial temporal sclerosis; SW slow waves; HASW high-amplitude slow waves; SPSW spiked slow waves; HASPSW high-amplitude spiked slow waves.

Table 1. Patients enrolled in the first study (Manganotti, 2008).

The good results we obtained (BOLD activations correlated to IEDs in 8/8 patients) allowed us to extend the study to 8 other patients (for a total of 16 patients), all with the same characteristics: focal epilepsy in which routine EEG recordings showed frequent focal IEDs manifesting as 5-6 Hz focal EEG activity (slow waves, slow spike waves, high-amplitude slow waves) over a few lateralized electrodes. The results did not change. MRI revealed a structural lesion in 4 patients: MTS in 2, tuberose sclerosis (TS) in 1; and hypothalamic hamartoma (HH) in 1. Three patients had cryptogenic and one nonlesional (idiopathic) epilepsy.

Standard EEG showed: focal sharp-wave activity in 1 patient (P15) with idiopathic epilepsy; high-amplitude slow-wave activity (or high-amplitude sharp waves) in 1 with TS (P12) and in 1 with HH (P14); spiked sharp waves in 1 with MTS (P10) and in 2 patients with cryptogenic epilepsy (P13 and P16); and high-amplitude spiked waves in 1 with MTS (P9) and in 1 with cryptogenic epilepsy (P11) (Table 2).

Patient	Type of epilepsy	Standard MRI findings	IED morphology	Irritative focus
9	Lesional	MTS	HASPSW	T8
10	Lesional	MTS	SPSW	F7-T3
11	Cryptogenic	Negative	HASPSW	F7-T3
12	Lesional	TS	HASW	P4
13	Cryptogenic	Negative	SPSW	T6
14	Lesional	HH	HASW	T4-T6
15	Idiopathic	Negative	SW	T3-T5
16	Cryptogenic	Negative	SPSW	F8-T4

Table 2. Characteristics of the 8 additional patients. MTS denotes mesial temporal sclerosis; TS tuberose sclerosis; HH: hypothalamic hamartoma.

6.2. Matherials and methods

6.2.1. EEG recordings and analysis

The EEG was acquired using a MR compatible EEG amplifier (SD MRI 32, Micromed, Treviso, Italy) and a cap providing 32 Ag/AgCl electrodes positioned according to a 10/20 system (impedance was kept below 10 kΩ). To remove pulse and movement artifacts during scanning two of these electrodes were used to record the electrocardiogram (ECG) and electromyogram (EMG). The EMG electrode was placed on the right abductor pollicis brevis (APB) muscle and the other (ECG) on the precordial area.

The reference was placed anterior to Fz, and the ground posterior to Fz as in other studies (Gonçalves et al. 2006; Avesani et al. 2008/a; Formaggio et al., 2008; Manganotti et al. 2008) using the same system. To ensure subjects' safety, the wires were carefully arranged to avoid loops and physical contact with the subject. To minimize the variability in the EEG artifacts due to the MR sequence and avoid wire movement caused by mechanical vibration the wires rested on foam pads.

EEG data were acquired at the rate of 1024 Hz using the software package SystemPlus (Micromed, Treviso, Italy). To avoid saturation, the EEG amplifier had a resolution of 22 bits with a range of ±25.6 mV. An anti-aliasing hardware band-pass filter was applied with a bandwidth between 0.15 and 269.5 Hz. Details of the EEG recording method are given in Bènar (Bènar et al, 2003). The EEG artifact induced by the gradient magnetic field was digitally removed off-line by an adaptive filter (Micromed). EEG artifacts associated with pulsatile blood flow were digitally removed off-line using a simple averaging procedure (Allen, 1998-2000). Subsequently a single electroencephalographer visually reviewed the filtered EEGs, and marked the time of onset and duration of each IED.

6.2.2. fMRI acquisition and analysis

Images were acquired on a 1.5 T MR scanner (Symphony, Siemens, Erlangen, Germany) equipped with EPI capability and a standard transient/receive (TR) head coil. At the start of each study, a T1-weighted anatomical MRI was acquired (192 slices; FOV = 256X256; scanning matrix 512X512; slice thickness 1 mm; sagittal slice orientation; echo time (TE) = 3ms; repetition time (TR) = 1990 ms).

All patients then underwent a 24-min fMRI recording session, after giving informed consent. BOLD fMRI data were acquired, using a standard gradient-echo (EPI) sequence, on the axial orientation, in 1 run of 8 minutes with the patient in the resting state, as described by the Kobayashi team (Kobayashi,2006) (voxel dimension 3x3x3 mm; 36 slices; matrix 64x64; TE = 50 ms, TR = 3.7 s; and slice thickness = 3 mm). At the onset of each fMRI acquisition, the scanner provided a trigger signal that was recorded by the EEG system and used as a volume marker.

For image processing and statistical analysis of the fMRI time series data we used BrainVoyager QX 1.9 software (*Brain Innovation, Maastricht, Netherlands*) running in windows VISTA enviroment. Pre-processing of the functional MRI included three-dimensional motion correction, slice scan time correction (linear interpolation), linear trend removal by temporal high-pass filtering (3 cycles in time course) and transformation into the Talairach coordinate space. Neither spatial nor temporal smoothing was used.

In each subject, activated voxels were identified with a single-subject general linear model (GLM) approach for time series data (Friston, 1995). To account for the hemodynamic delay, the boxcar waveform representing the rest and task conditions was convolved with an empirical hemodynamic response function (Friston, 1998).

A t statistic was used to determine significance on a voxel-by-voxel basis and correlation values were transformed into a normal distribution (Z statistic). The results were displayed on parametric statistical maps in which the pixel Z value is expressed on a colorimetric scale. We identified the single region of condition-associated BOLD signal changes with a statistical threshold based on the amplitude ($p<0.05$) and extent of the regions of activation. The location of voxels with maximal signal increase was expressed in terms of x, y, and z in the Talairach space, and activation volumes were expressed in terms of number of activated voxels. Positive BOLD-fMRI responses were defined as activations. Significant responses were defined as almost five contiguous voxels with $p<0.05$ over at least two contiguous slices (Krakow 1999 and 2001; Salek-Haddadi 2006) in 2D-reconstruction. The anatomic localization of BOLD responses was determined by co-registration of the anatomic data and statistical t maps.

We analyzed the extent and maximum fMRI response for each study, considering all areas with significative activations. We also determined the locations of maximum activation based on the maximum peak response (maximum t value).

6.3. Results

In all patients, EEG showed unilateral focal activity during the EEG-fMRI session. IEDs recorded inside the scanner had a localization, amplitude and morphology similar to those seen in the previous routine EEG recordings. EEG recordings showed focal high-amplitude slow waves in 4 patients (P1, P6, P12 and P14), and slow-wave discharges over the temporal electrodes in the other 3 patients (P2, P4 and P15). In 1 patient (P7) slow-wave activity was detected in the extratemporal (F7) region. In the patient with a cavernoma (P3), in 1 with MTS

(P10), and in 2 patients with cryptogenic epilepsy (P13 and P16), focal EEG activity was characterized by focal slow-spiked wave activity, reaching maximal amplitude over the left temporal electrodes (T5). In 1 patient (P5) slow-spiked waves were detected in the extratemporal region (left occipital region). The EEG tracings also showed high-amplitude spiked slow-wave activity in 3 patients (P8, P9 and P11): in the right temporal region in 2 (P8 and P9) and in the left fronto-temporal region in 1 patient (P11).

The mean frequency was 2.4 IEDs per minute (SD 0.17) for the first 8 patients and 2.495 for the second 8 patients, thus confirming sample homogeneity.

In all 8 patients from the first study and in 7/8 from the second study, fMRI analysis showed, in 2-D reconstruction, significant focal BOLD activation in a single activated area related to the EEG irritative focus (Tables 3 and 4). This activation was considered significant (Krakow, 1999) because it was identified in two contiguous MRI slices.

Patient	IEDs/24 min	IEDs/min	BOLD activation in 2D reconstruction	No. of slices
1	61	2.54	Left mesial temporal lobe	2
2	55	2.29	Left mesial temporal lobe	2
3	54	2.25	Left superior temporal lobe – neocortical region	3
4	58	2.41	Right mesial temporal lobe	2
5	64	2.66	Left occipital lobe-calcarin cortex	2
6	51	2.13	Right superior temporal lobe	2
7	58	2.41	Left frontal lobe	2
8	62	2.58	Right superior temporal lobe	2

Table 3. Number of IEDs revealed on EEG during recording and BOLD activation in 2D reconstruction of fMRI, with number of contiguous activated slices.

Patient	IEDs/24 min	IEDs/min	BOLD activation in 2D reconstruction	No. of slices
9	57	2.38	Left mesial temporal lobe	3
10	57	2.38	Left mesial temporal lobe	3
11	59	2.45	Left supplementary motor cortex	5
12	62	2.59	Right parietal lobe	3
13	64	2.66	Right mesial temporal lobe	2
14	65	2.70	Right mesial temporal lobe	2
15	53	2.20	====	0
16	63	2.60	Left mesial temporal lobe	2

Table 4. Number of IEDs revealed on EEG during recording and BOLD activation in 2D reconstruction of fMRI, with number of contiguous activated slices, in the second study of 8 patients.

This result was confirmed with analysis of 3D reconstruction of fMRI: in all 8 patients from the first study (Manganotti, 2008) and in 7/8 from the second study, fMRI BOLD activation corresponded to the irritative focus on standard EEG recordings (Tables 5 and 6).

Patient	No of voxels	Corresponding area in 3D reconstruction
1	177	Left cerebrum, limbic lobe, parahippocampal gyrus, **Brodmann area 34**
2	522	Left cerebrum, limbic lobe, parahippocampal gyrus, **Brodmann area 30**
3	540	Left cerebrum, temporal lobe, inferior temporal gyrus, **Brodmann area 20**
4	175	Right cerebrum, limbic lobe, parahippocampal gyrus, **Brodmann area 28**
5	1227	Left cerebrum occipital lobe, lingual gyrus, **Brodmann area 18**
6	364	Right cerebrum, temporal lobe, transverse temporal gyrus, **Brodmann area 42**
7	442	Left cerebrum, frontal lobe, precentral gyrus, **Brodmann area 6**
8	422	Right cerebrum, temporal lobe, middle temporal gyrus, **Brodmann area 21**

Table 5. Number of activated voxels, and localization, according to the Talairach system, of activated regions in 3D reconstruction, of the 8 patients from the first study (Manganotti, 2008).

Patient	No. of voxels	Activation in 3D reconstruction
9	368	1) Right cerebrum, temporal lobe, superior temporal gyrus **Brodmann area 38** 2) Right cerebrum, frontal lobe, mesial frontal region **Brodman area 10**
10	350	Left cerebrum, temporal lobe, fusiform gyrus **Brodmann area 20**
11	322	Left cerebrum, frontal lobe, supplementary motor cortex **Brodmann area 6**
12	52	Right cerebrum, parietal lobe, precuneus **Brodmann area 7**
13	256	Right cerebrum, temporal lobe, superior temporal gyrus **Brodmann area 38**
14	200	Right cerebrum, anterior cingulate, limbic lobe **Brodmann area 32**
15	0	=====
16	150	Right cerebrum, parahippocampal gyrus, limbic lobe **Brodmann area 34**

Table 6. Number of activated voxels, and localization, according to the Talairach system, of activated regions in 3D reconstruction, of the 8 patients from the second study.

6.3.1. Temporal lobe activation

Focal BOLD signal changes in 11 patients reached statistical significance in the temporal regions. In 10 patients (4 of which with MTS [P1, P4, P9, and P10]; 1 with HH [P14]; 3 with cryptogenic epilepsy [P2, P13, and P16]; in 2 of the 4 with idiopathic epilepsy [P6 and P8]), the significant BOLD changes were located in the mesial temporal lobe and in the neocortical regions (laterally and posteriorly to the resection margins) in the 1 patient with a cavernoma (P3).

An interesting case of surgically treated mesial temporal sclerosis involved P9. Of Moroccan origin, he has suffered from focal seizures since the age of 6 years, with loss of consciousness and oral and motor automatisms of the legs (pedaling) and arms, preceded by an epigastric aura, lasting 1 minute and resistant to therapy. On MRI, right mesial temporal sclerosis (MTS) was detected (fig.3). Standard EEG demonstrated an interictal focus in the right temporal region. The seizures first occurred rarely but then increased in frequency with time, eventually manifesting in "clusters" of 10-15 seizures every 1 to 2 months. Auras occurred every 2 weeks. Video-EEG demonstrated the same abnormal activity in the right temporal region, with an ictal event manifesting with the same characteristics. The hypothesis was that the seizures arose in an epileptogenic area related to the known MTS and then spread anteriorly to the right mesial frontal region (cause of motor manifestation). EEG-fMRI recording session identified an interictal slow wave activity in right temporal region (T4-T6), with a following diffusion both to contralateral region and to right frontal region (fig. 4). Two significant activations were detected (figg. 5-6): one in the right mesial temporal region (Brodmann area 38) and one in the right mesial frontal region (Brodmann area 10). Also in this case, BOLD activations were concordant with focal IEDs and with clinical syndrome. On subsequent analysis with invasive techniques (SEEG), the origin of seizure in an epileptogenic zone correlated with MTS was confirmed, with spread to the right mesial frontal region. The study also confirmed the co-localization between EEG and fMRI data. He was surgically treated and is now seizure free.

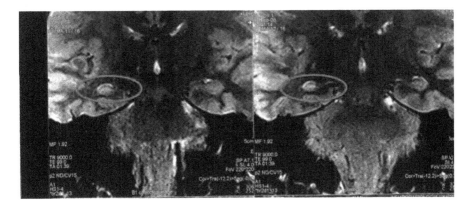

Figure 3. Right mesial temporal sclerosis (MTS) in Patient n. 9

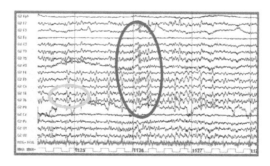

EEG recorded during scanning session (monopolar montage)

Irritative focus

Contralateral diffusion

Figure 4. Patient n. 9. Focal IEDs in right temporal region, with following diffusion both to contralateral region and to right frontal region

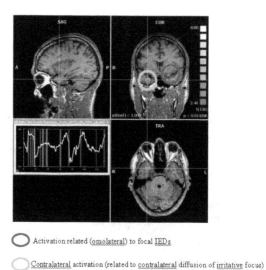

Activation related (omolateral) to focal IEDs

Contralateral activation (related to contralateral diffusion of irritative focus)

Figure 5. Patient n. 9. Focal IEDs correlated BOLD activations in mesial right temporal region, with following diffusion to contralateral region

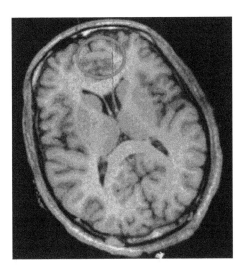

Figure 6. Patient n. 9. Focal IEDs correlated BOLD activation in right mesial frontal region

Another case involved a young man (P14) affected with gelastic seizures due to a hypothalamic hamartoma and manifesting since he was 2 years old. They were well defined: dissociated deviation of the eyes (the left eye toward the right and the right eye upwards) or associated deviation of both eyes upwards, followed by right head deviation, absent facial expression, and asymmetric smile. Often, an aura (tingling in the left temporal region) would precede the seizures, with concurrent rubor. The patient attempted to speak but was impeded by fixed smiling. The episode frequency was very high (up to 5 seizures/day). Over time, the syndrome worsened, with falls and subsequent injuries. SEEG confirmed an epileptogenic zone inside the hamartoma, with spread to the right mesial temporal region during the seizures. EEG-fMRI detected a significant BOLD activation in the limbic lobe (anterior cingulate), substantiating the anatomic-clinical correlation suggested by seizures and EEG.

This case parallels recently published findings on the networks involved in seizure generation in hypothalamic hamartoma (Kokkinos, 2012). EEG-fMRI was performed in 2 adult patients with hypothalamic hamartoma, the one with predominantly gelastic seizures and the other with complex partial but no typical gelastic seizures. Ictal and interictal analysis of the patient with gelastic seizures revealed involvement of the hypothalamic hamartoma, the cingulate gyrus, the precuneus and prefrontal cortex. The interictal analysis of the patient with complex partial seizures showed BOLD signal changes over the temporal lobes, the base of the frontal lobe, the precuneus and prefrontal cortex but not the hypothalamic hamartoma. It was presumed that the differences in the neural networks implicated may have accounted for the differences in the clinical manifestation of seizures owing to the tumor.

Other interesting cases are cryptogenic (P2, P13) and idiophatic forms (P6, P8, P15), all characterized by atypical absences and vagal symptomatology. In patient n. 2, focal IEDs (fig.

7) were recorded in left temporal region and focal IEDs correlated BOLD activation (fig. 8) was detected in mesial left temporal region, in limbic lobe. In patient n. 6 focal IEDs were recorded in right temporal region, with a characteristic phase reversal in T4 (fig. 9), and focal IEDs correlated BOLD activation was detected in Brodam area 42 (fig. 10). In patient n. 8, focal IEDs were recorded in right temporal region (fig. 11) and focal IEDs correlated BOLD activation was detected in Brodman area 21 (fig. 12).

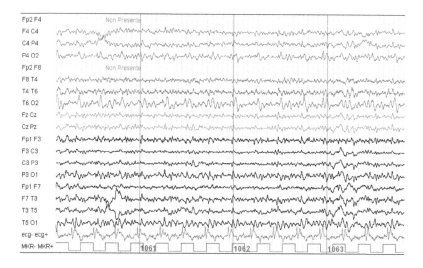

Figure 7. Patient n. 2 (cryptogenic epilepsy). Focal IEDs in left temporal region during scanning session

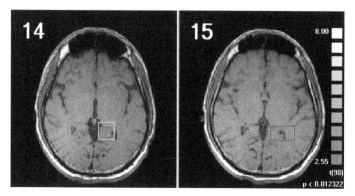

Figure 8. Patient n. 2. Focal IEDs correlated BOLD activations in left mesial temporal lobe

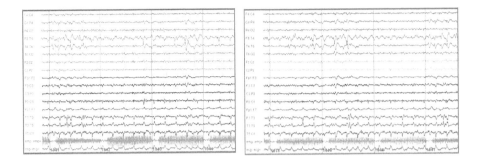

Figure 9. Patient n. 6. Focal IEDs in right temporal lobe with phase reversal in T4

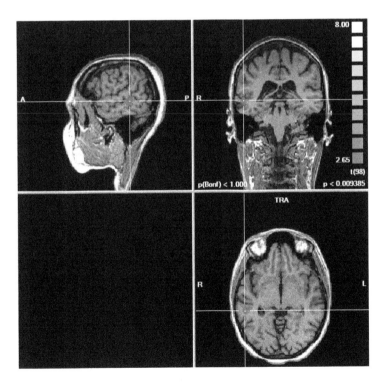

Figure 10. Patient n. 6. Focal IEDs correlated activation in transverse temporal gyrus, Brodmann area 42

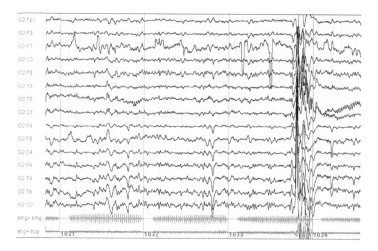

Figure 11. Patient n. 8. Focal IEDs in right temporal region

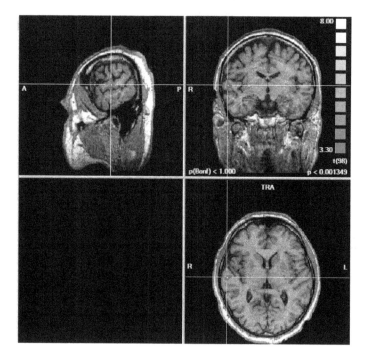

Figure 12. Patient n.8. Focal IEDs correlated BOLD activation in middle temporal gyrus, Brodmann area 21

6.3.2. Extratemporal activation

In our series, fMRI showed extratemporal activation in 4 patients: the left occipital lobe (P5); the left frontal lobe (P7); the left supplementary motor cortex (P11); and the right parietal lobe (P12). In all four cases there was a correlation between BOLD activation and IEDs and with clinical syndromes as well. This correlation is relevant to the discussion about the technique's sensitivity in revealing activation in extratemporal regions.

A rare case (P5) involved non ketotic hyperglycemia (NKH)-induced seizures occurring in the left occipital lobe studied by EEG-fMRI (Del Felice, 2009). These seizures usually occur in the frontal regions and cause motor ictal syndromes, whereas occipital seizures have been described in very rare situations. Cases of NKH presenting as hemichorea or hemianopia have also been reported. Seven such patients (Seo, 2003; Raghavendra, 2007) were studied by standard MRI transient T_2-weighted and fluid-attenuated inversion recovery (FLAIR). Subcortical hypointensity with or without abnormalities in the occipital overlying cortex or striatal nuclei was documented in occipital seizures associated with NKH. A single case investigated by Tc-99m HMPAO SPECT (Wang, 2005) showed occipital hyperperfusion during seizure recurrence and hypoperfusion during the interictal state.

Our patient (P5) was a 50-year-old woman admitted to hospital after repeated emergency room visits because of visual disturbances and left-sided headache. On clinical examination, she was obese and had a right-sided homonymous hemianopia. Her medical history was unremarkable, except for hypertension and a 15-kg weight gain during the past 12 months. She had no history of migraine, epilepsy or neurological disorders. Two days before admission she reported a short-lasting episode of visual disturbance (distortion). A few hours later, she noted diplopia when looking to the right, with image distortion in the right visual field and intermittent right-sided hemianopia, lasting several minutes, elicited by looking to the right or by fixation. The episodes were accompanied by a left-sided throbbing headache but no other autonomic symptoms (i.e., nausea or vomiting). No language disturbance was reported. She was presented to the emergency room.

On neurological examination, a right-sided homonymous hemianopia was noted. A standard computed tomography (CT) scan of the brain and an ophthalmologic exam were negative. She was discharged with a diagnosis of migraine with aura and started on antiplatelet therapy, with the recommendation to undergo out-patient visual field analysis.

Two days later, she was admitted to our ward owing to the persistence of symptoms, including a transient conjugated deviation of the eyes and the head to the right. On that occasion, which lasted less than 1 minute, the patient did not lose consciousness and referred seeing red flashing lights in her right visual field. Standard EEG performed immediately thereafter showed multiple clinical-EEG seizures during a prolonged recording, with spiked slow waves originating from the left posterior region, and with bilateral diffusion (fig. 13). Laboratory data on admission revealed hyperglycemia (14.5 mm/L to 261 mg/dL) with a serum osmolarity of 333 mmol/kg, and glycosilated hemoglobin of 10.5%. Urine analysis was negative for ketone bodies but was strongly positive for glycosuria (>1 g/dL) and microalbuminuria (up to 6 mg/24 h). A brain MRI scan with and without gadolinium, an MR angiography, and a 3T brain

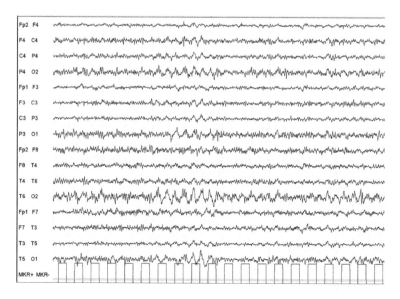

Figure 13. Patient n. 5. Standard EEG tracing during clinical seizures. Spiked slow waves on posterior regions (O1 and O2).

MRI were normal. Tc-99m hexamethylpropylene amine oxime (HMPAO) single-photon-emission computed tomography (SPECT), during which no clinical seizures were reported, showed non-significant hypocaptation over the posterior regions bilaterally.

On continuous EEG-fMRI a few days later, no clinical or EEG manifestations of ictal events occurred, but interictal spiked slow wave discharges (IEDs) with localization, amplitude and morphology similar to those previously recorded on routine EEG (fig. 13) were noted. A slow-spiked wave on the left occipital (O1) channel was detected. The mean frequency was 2.4 IEDs per minute. Functional MRI analysis showed significant focal BOLD activation in a single area related to the EEG paroxysmal activity. In a 3D reconstruction using the Talairach system (fig. 14), focal significant BOLD activation based on the EEG-related protocol was identified in Brodmann area 18 (grey matter of the left cerebrum occipital lobe and lingual gyrus). During her hospital stay, she was started on carbamazepine (200 mg/daily, up to 800 mg t. d.), with only partial benefit in frequency and intensity of symptoms. Since her glycemia was still uncontrolled (250 mg/dL), she was started on insulin therapy. Over the following 2 weeks, seizures and hyperglycemia both progressively decreased. On the basis of a possible diagnosis of NKH-induced seizures, carbamazepine was tapered, without the reappearance of symptoms. Serial EEG showed a decrease in epileptic activity (sharp waves) with persistent bilateral slowing. A few weeks later, insulin therapy was replaced with oral antidiabetics. One year later, the patient was seizure free, with a normal EEG. Following the loss of 18 kg, the oral antidiabetics were tapered, with good control of serum glucose and HbA1 values.

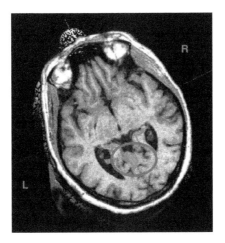

Figure 14. Patient n. 5. 3D fMRI-BOLD activation in Brodmann area 18.

A BOLD occipital activation in patients referring visual symptoms has been reported, confirming the involvement of visual functional areas in the occipital lobes: Brodmann areas 19 and 37 in reported cases of fixation sensitivity occipital spiking (Iannetti et al., 2002; Avesani, 2008/b) or the left occipital lobe in cases of cryptogenic and symptomatic (cortical malformation) occipital epilepsy (Salek-Haddadi et al., 2006). In our patient, an analogous BOLD activation was elicited by the NKH. Hyperglycemia may induce paroxysmal activity in brain areas more susceptible to metabolic changes – the occipital lobe in this case - with an analogous pattern of activation of self-sustained focal discharges. Neuroimaging, in this case fMRI-EEG co-registration, pointed to a change in blood volume in the involved posterior areas.

In the patient (P7) in whom fMRI revealed BOLD activation in the left frontal region (Brodmann area 6), standard EEG showed a left fronto-temporal irritative focus characterized by frequent slow-spiked waves. A recent polygraphic study (recorded during stage I and II non-rapid-eye-movement [NREM] sleep) showed polymorphic slow waves (theta-delta) in the left frontal regions, with phase inversion at F7 and without spread. These findings suggested that the patient was a good candidate for an EEG-fMRI study. During the EEG-fMRI sessions, we confirmed the fMRI activation area within the precentral gyrus.

Patient no. 11, a young woman, illustrates an interesting case of frontal lobe epilepsy characterized by focal seizures, with speech arrest and right arm clonus followed by generalization (Borelli, 2010), where, as reported elsewhere (So, 1998; Westmoreland, 1998), scalp EEG is often ambiguous because it is poorly sensitive to deep generators on the mesial surface of the frontal lobe. Also in this instance, EEG-fMRI effectively identified the interictal focus.

According to a detailed account by relatives, the events took the form of sudden episodes of speech arrest lasting from a few seconds up to several minutes, without any warning sensation. The patient reported she was able to move, understand and write properly during the ictal phase (sometimes writing a note to her husband that she was unable to speak). No clonic movements or orofacial automatisms were experienced at this early stage. Usually, an event did not progress any further and the patient was able to fully recollect the episode. Sometimes an episode was followed by clonic jerking over the right side of the face and arms with occasional, generalized tonic-clonic seizures. The seizure frequency was weekly despite polytherapy. The 3T MRI was normal. She reported no febrile seizures nor having sustained significant head injuries. Pregnancy, delivery and developmental milestones were unremarkable, as was the remainder of her medical history. Trials with various antiepileptic drugs (first with dintoine, then carbamazepine, and then fenobarbital) were unsuccessful. She was admitted to an intensive care unit for a status epilepticus and begun on valproate and lamotrigine.

Interictal scalp EEG showed frequent generalized high-amplitude (2 to 3 Hz) spiked slow-wave discharges. There was an inconstant, mild amplitude prevalence over the left hemisphere electrodes (F7-T3).

During a conventional scalp EEG recording, she complained of a brief episode of speech arrest associated with an EEG pattern characterized by diffuse spike and wave discharges (fig. 15). This event was witnessed by a neurologist from our ward who was aware of the patient's clinical history. He noted that the patient had a brief inability to speak (a few seconds) during which she waved her hands to attract his attention. There were no clonic movements, and after regaining speech, she accurately described the event. Three-hour video-EEG monitoring during a day of seizure clustering recorded no usual events. On the basis of these elements, a diagnosis of generalized epilepsy was also made in another hospital.

The clinical syndrome suggested involvement of the left supplementary motor area (SMA) with spread to the primary motor area. EEG -fMRI recording session confirmed the same pattern EEG identified by standard EEG (fig. 16) and following analysis showed prominent BOLD activation over the left SMA during the high-amplitude spiked slow-wave discharges compared to the rest state (Fig. 17). According to the Duncan criteria, such an activation pattern is reproducible since it was present in two contiguous slices (Duncan, 1999). The statistical significance of the activation was $p < 0.0028$ even after FDR correction. More activations were found in the contralateral SMA and homolateral motor strip as well. No significant deactivation areas or thalamic involvement (activation or deactivation) were found. The patient was referred to a level II epilepsy surgery center for presurgical work-up, including long-term video-EEG monitoring, but she refused further testing.

The speech arrest noted in this patient is an epileptic feature usually related to involvement of the supplementary motor cortex over either the dominant or the non-dominant hemisphere. A bilateral spike and wave discharge pattern (secondary bilateral synchrony) is often detected in frontal-lobe epilepsy, particularly if the generator is deep, for instance, over the mesial surface of the frontal lobe (So, 1998; Westmoreland, 1998). In the presurgical work-up for epilepsy surgery, such a scalp EEG pattern certainly raises questions about the origin of the focal epilepsy especially when conventional MRI is negative. In the latter case, more investigations are usually obtained to guide depth electrode placement for invasive EEG. Ictal SPECT and interictal PET are commonly used for this purpose, but they are expensive, difficult to interpret, and usually provide regional rather than local data. In addition, if the ictal event is

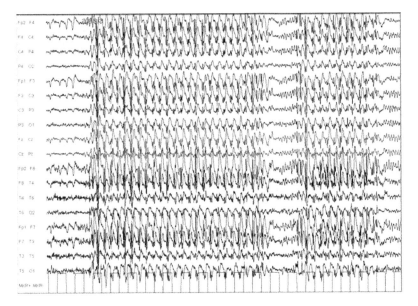

Figure 15. Patient n. 11. Ictal EEG during a brief speech arrest episode ("Afasia" marks the beginning of the speech impairment).

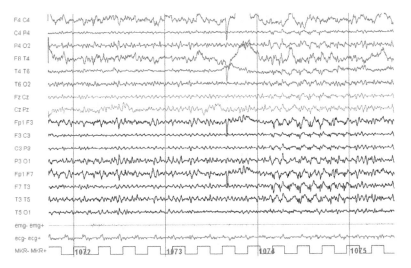

Figure 16. Patient n.11. EEG recorded during the fMRI acquisition showing generalized high amplitude spiked slow wave discharges, prevalent on left fronto-temporal regions.

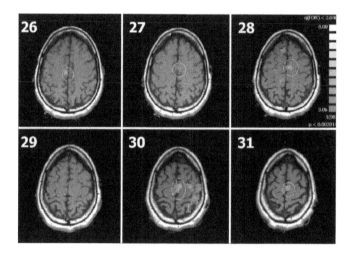

Figure 17. Patient n. 11. The EEG-fMRI shows a clear-cut activation of the left (radiological convention) Supplementary Motor Area (SMA) and on the contralateral SMA on a lesser degree. Spread over the left motor strip is also evident.

brief, SPECT may yield false negatives due to incorrect timing of the tracer injection (Salmenpera, 2005; Devous, 1998). The use of radioactive substances also raises safety issues.

A relatively new tool to obtain localizing data on the basis of EEG changes, EEG-fMRI is safe for the patient and relatively inexpensive (Al Asmi, 2003; Di Bonaventura, 2006). As our knowledge about the technique increases, it is gaining acceptance in the study of focal nonlesional epilepsy and presurgical work-up, as reported by Moeller et al. and Zijlmans et al. (Devous, 1998; Moeller, 2009). Nonetheless, few studies to date have applied EEG-fMRI in patients with secondary bilateral synchrony, except for one by Aghakhani (Aghakhani, 2006) involving 11 patients with such an EEG pattern, with a variable activation-deactivation pattern including thalamic involvement in 6 out of 11 (55%). The clinical seizure pattern and the MRI findings were variable.

In our patient, EEG-fMRI revealed the origin of the epileptiform discharges, including the spread over the homolateral motor strip, which was highly consistent with the patient's clinical features (speech arrest followed by clonic jerks over right half of the face and right arm), whereas 3T MRI and conventional interictal scalp EEG were useless in this regard. Some involvement of the contralateral SMA was also detected but its significance is less clear: it may have been the result of a transcallosal spread from the left SMA or simply an imperfect spatial resolution of the technique. In contrast with Aghakhani (Aghakhani, 2006) in our case no thalamic changes were seen.

Unfortunately, our localizing hypothesis could not be proved by invasive EEG and postsurgical outcome since the patient refused surgical treatment. Nonetheless, this patient suggests that, in the presurgical work up for epilepsy, EEG-fMRI may be considered a useful tool to generate a localizing hypothesis to be tested with invasive recording also in patients with focal epilepsy and bilateral slow spiked-wave discharges on EEG (secondary bilateral synchrony) and negative MRI. The recording of ictal EEG demonstrates that the slow waves we triggered in our study were irritative and not lesional.

7. Conclusions

The main finding in our EEG-fMRI study of patients with partial epilepsy is that the focal interictal slow-wave activity was invariably associated with increased focal fMRI-BOLD activation responses in a spatially related brain area. Our study extends current knowledge on epileptic foci localization and confirms previous reports suggesting that EEG-fMRI BOLD activation associated with modeled slow activity might have a role in localizing the epilepto-genic region, even in the absence of clear interictal spikes (Laufs, 2006; Avesani, 2008/a).

All the patients with partial epilepsy we enrolled in this study had frequent interictal focal slow-wave activity on standard EEG. In all continuous EEG-fMRI recording sessions, after fMRI artifact removal, we obtained good quality EEG that allowed us to detect spontaneous IEDs and analyze the related fMRI BOLD activation. The EEG recording left the quality of the fMRI data almost undistorted, and the focal activity seen in the concurrent EEG was associated, in 15 of 16 patients enrolled, with a focal increase in the MRI signal in all patients. In their focal distribution, these BOLD activations resembled the focal IEDs seen on routine scalp EEG and EEG recorded during EEG-fMRI sessions.

An interesting finding came from the patients with lesional epilepsy. These patients, whose standard MRI documented a lesion and whose standard EEG identified an irritative focus, are ideal candidates for verifying a possible spatial relationship between the epileptogenic and the irritative focus (Ebersole, 1991; Benbadis, 1996).

In the patient who had undergone surgery to remove a cavernoma (P3), the EEG-fMRI study, by localizing the irritative focus and linking it to fMRI as an "active state", showed a significant BOLD activation signal closely related to the poro-encephalic cavity (a residual of previous treatment). Although this focal BOLD activation presumably arose from a blood vessel (residual cavernoma), it was undoubtedly obtained by a protocol study linking an active fMRI state to IEDs on EEG. To clarify the relationship, we decided to progressively test the specificity to a very high level ($p < 0.0001$), as demonstrated in the iconography. Even with these high specificity values, the BOLD activation in that site persisted.

Another new finding is the BOLD activation we detected on fMRI in the patients with MTS. In contrast to others who studied a series of patients with MTS (5 studied with continuous co-registration) (Al Asmi, 2003) and found no significant activation, we detected significant BOLD activation in 4 patients (P1, P4, P9 and P10). These results suggest a possible role of simulta-neous EEG-fMRI in disclosing focal activation in the mesial temporal cortex. This cortical area is notoriously difficult to study with standard methods because the deep localization of the irritative area often makes spikes smoother and therefore harder to recognize on recordings from standard EEG scalp electrodes than in SEEG. Hence, IEDs presenting as slow-wave discharges could be useful in determining significant BOLD activation in a corresponding area, as previously suggested by Laufs et al. (Laufs, 2006).

Useful information that may help us to understand BOLD responses in various forms of epilepsy came also from studying activation in extratemporal IEDs. In the patients with extratemporal discharges (P5, P7, P11, and P12), we noted a good correlation between the clinical polygraphic data and BOLD activation during fMRI. No significant difference was found between activation in the frontal or the occipital lobe. In both regions, BOLD activation increased after focal IEDs. One patient (P11) demonstrated the usefulness of EEG-fMRI, especially when scalp EEG is ambiguous because it is poorly sensitive to detect deep generators on the mesial surface of the frontal lobe, and confirmed that the slow waves were irritative and not lesional.

The reason for such good results (15/16 activations -- significant concordance between EEG and fMRI data) is open to question. The most plausible reason is that during enrolment, to obtain the largest possible percentage of activations, patients were explicitly selected whose standard EEGs showed a high IED firing rate confirmed on EEG during the scanning session. The mean frequency of IEDs in the 15 patients was about 2/min, considerably higher than the 1 IED per minute Duncan considered as the minimum to obtain a focal BOLD activation (Krakow, 1999). Collectively, these findings confirm the importance of IED firing rates in EEG-fMRI.

Perhaps the most interesting finding in this study was that morphology seemed less important than IED firing rates in triggering EEG-fMRI-BOLD activation: 8 of the 16 patients had pure slow waves on standard EEG (4 with high amplitude and 4 with a normal voltage) and 7 had slow spike-wave discharges (4 with high amplitude and 3 with normal voltage); 1 patient (P10) had a focus of normal amplitude, sometimes pure, sometimes with spiked morphology. There were no differences in BOLD activation between the two groups.

Although these slow spike-wave discharges might have originated from a spike focus smoothed by filtering (unlikely because EEG detected the same IEDs before the patients entered the magnet room), there was no difference in the statistical significance of BOLD activation between the two groups. Specifically, slow spike-wave IEDs were no more efficient than slow-wave IEDs in eliciting significant BOLD activation. Hence, it was agreed as previously suggested (Laufs, 2006/a; Avesani, 2008/a) that slow-wave IEDs, like spikes, could elicit a significant increase in cerebral blood flow in a spatially related brain area.

The study also suggests that voltage might have a minor role in determining BOLD activation: in this small study sample there were no differences in BOLD activations between IEDs with high-amplitude (9 patients) and those with normal amplitude slow waves (7 patients).

The significant concordance between EEG and fMRI data, and the absence of multiple activation areas in particular, depended on the high specificity threshold the study design envisaged. In designing this study, only the single activation with the strongest specificity was maintained so that we could verify whether this activation, and this activation alone, coincided with the epileptic focus previously documented by standard EEG and used as a paradigm for the activation-state during the fMRI analysis.

Given the criticism raised against the use of EEG-fMRI instead of other techniques such as EEG-source analysis in the presurgical work-up (Elshoff, 2012), a possible objection to the conclusions we draw could derive from our decision to include only a well-defined sample of patients, all characterized by a focus with a high firing rate, without evidence of the same result in other patients with low firing rate foci (being the most frequent among patients affected by focal drug-resistant epilepsy of surgical interest. We reply that this study was the first approach to investigating interictal slow-wave foci. This will be addressed in a future study in order to validate the technique in patients with slow-wave interictal activity with a low firing rate focus.

At the moment, the complete EEG-fMRI concordance achieved in this study suggests that slow-wave IEDs, even without spikes, may be useful in activating fMRI BOLD responses during the presurgical, noninvasive evaluation of patients with partial drug-resistant seizures.

Acknowledgements

The authors wish to thank:

- Prof. Bernardo Dalla Bernardina, Dp of Life and Reproduction Sciences, University of Verona

- Dr. Giuseppe Moretto and Dr. Tiziano Zanoni, Dp of Neurological Sciences, Civil Hospital of Verona, Dp of Neurological Sciences, Civil Hospital of Verona

- Prof. Nicolò Rizzuto, Dp of Neurological, Neuropsychological, Morphological and Movement Sciences, University of Verona

- Dr. Paolo Manganotti, Dr. Luigi Giuseppe Bongiovanni, Dr. Paolo Borelli, Dr. Alessandra Del Felice, dott. Emanuela Formaggio, dott. Silvia Francesca Storti, Dp of Neurological, Neuropsychological, Morphological and Movement Sciences, University of Verona, Dp of Neurological, Neuropsychological, Morphological and Movement Sciences, University of Verona for their collaboration

- Prof. Roberto Pozzi Mucelli, Dr.ssa Anna Gasparini and Dr. Roberto Cerini, Dp of Radiology University of Verona

Author details

Mirko Avesani[1], Silvia Giacopuzzi[2] and Antonio Fiaschi[1]

1 University of Verona, Department of Neurological, Neuropsychological, Morphological and Movement Sciences, Italy

2 University of Verona, Department of Life and Reproduction Sciences, Italy

References

[1] Aghakhani et al. fMRI activation during spike wave discharges in idiopatic general-
     ized epilepsy. Brain, 2004; 127: 1127-1144

[2] Aghakhani et al. The role of periventricular nodular heterotopia in epileptogenesis.
     Brain, 2005; 128: 641-651

[3] Aghakhani et al. Cortical and thalamic fMRI responses in partial epilepsy with focal
     and bilateral synchronous spikes. Clin Neurophysiol 2006;117:177–91.

[4] Archer et al. fMRI "deactivation" of the posterior cingulate during generalized spike
     and wave. Neuroimage. 2003;20:1915–1922.

[5] Al-Asmi et al. fMRI activation in continuous and spike-triggered EEG-fMRI studies
     of epileptic spikes. Epilepsia, 2003; 44: 1328-1339.

[6] Allen et al. Identification of EEG events in the MR scanner: the problem of pulse arti-
     fact and a method for its subtraction. Neuroimage, 1998; 8: 229-239.

[7] Allen et al. A method for removing imaging artefact from continuous EEG recorded
     during functional MRI. Neuroimage, 2000; 12:230-239.

[8] Archer et al. fMRI "deactivation" of the posterior cingulate during generalized spike
     and wave. Neuroimage. 2003;20:1915–1922.

[9] Archer et al. Spike-triggered fMRI in reading epilepsy: involvement of left frontal
     cortex working memory areas. Neurology, 2003; 60: 415-421

[10] Avesani et al. Continuous EEG-fMRI in pre surgical evaluation of a patient affected
     by symptomatic seizures: BOLD activation linked to interictal epileptiform discharg-
     es caused by cavernoma. The Neuroradiology Journal, 2008/a; 21: 183-191.

[11] Avesani et al. fMRI in epilepsy with spike and wave activity evoked by eye closure:
     different BOLD activation in a patient with idiopathic partial epilepsy with occipital
     spikes and a control group. Neuroradiol. J., 2008/b; 21:159—165.

[12] Bagshaw et al. EEG-fMRI of focal epileptic spikes: analysis with multiple haemodya-
     mic functions and comparision with gadolinium-enhanced MR angiograms. Human
     Brain Mapping, 2004; 22: 179-192

[13] Bagshaw et al. Correspondence between EEG-fMRI and EEG dipole localization of
     interictal discharges in focal epilepsy. Neuroimage, 2006; 30: 417-425

[14] Benar et al. Quality of EEG in simultaneous EEG-fMRI for epilepsy. Clin Neurophy-
     siol, 2003; 114: 569-580.

[15] Benar et al. EEG-fMRI of epileptic spikes. Concordance with EEG source localization
     and intracranial EEG. Neuroimage, 2006; 30: 1161-1170

[16]   Berns. Functional neuroimaging. Life Sci. 1999; 65: 2531-2540.

[17]   Bernasconi et al. Proton magnetic resonance spectroscopic imaging suggests progressive neuronal damage in human temporal lobe epilepsy. Prog. Brain Res, 2002; 135: 297-304

[18]   Binder et al. Determination of language dominance using functional MRI: a comparision with Wada test. Neurology, 1996; 46: 978-984

[19]   Boly et al. Intrinsic brain activity in altered states of consciousness: how conscious is the default mode of brain function? Ann N Y Acad Sci. 2008;1129:119–129.

[20]   Boor et al. EEG-related functional MRI in beningn childhood epilepsy with centrotemporal spikes. Epilepsia, 2003; 44: 688-692

[21]   Borelli et al. EEG-fMRI as an useful tool to detect epileptic foci associated with secondary

[22]   bilateral synchrony. Seizure, 2010; 19:605-608.

[23]   Cavanna. The precuneuos and consciousness. CNS Spectr. 2007;12:545–552.

[24]   Cavanna et al . The precuneus: a review of its functional anatomy and behavioural correlates. Brain. 2006;129:564–583.

[25]   David et al. Identifying neural drivers with functional MRI: an electrophysiological validation. PLoS Biol. 2008;23:2683–2697.

[26]   Del Felice et al. EEG-fMRI coregistration in non ketotic hyperglicemic occipital seizures. Epilepsy Research, 2009;85(2-3):321-324

[27]   De Tiège et al. Impact of interictal epileptic activity on normal brain function in epileptic encephalopathy: an EEG-fMRI study. Epilepsy Behav. 2007;11:460–465.

[28]   Devous et al. SPECT brain imaging in epilepsy: a meta-analysis. J Nucl Med 1998;39:285–93.

[29]   Devous et al. Single-photon emission computed tomography in neurotherapeutic. NeuroRx 2005, 2: 237-249

[30]   Di Bonaventura. EEG/fMRI study of ictal and interictal epileptic activity: methodological issues and future perspectives in clinical practice. Epilepsia, 2006; 47, Suppl. 5: 52-58.

[31]   Duncan et al. Imaging and epilepsy. Brain 1997; 120: 339-377

[32]   Dupon et al. Bilateral hemispheric alteration of memory processes in right medial temporal lobe epilepsy. J Neurol Neurosurg Psych, 2002; 73: 478-485

[33]   Elshoff et al. The value of EEG-fMRI and EEG source analysis in the presurgical set-up of children with refractory focal epilepsy. Epilepsia, 2012; 53: 1597-1606.

[34] Engel et al. Comparative localization of epileptic foci in partial epilepsy by PCT and EEG. Ann Neurol 1982; 12: 529-537.

[35] Engel et al. Local cerebral metabolism during partial seizures. Neurology, 1983; 33: 400-413

[36] Faymonville et al. Functional neuroanatomy of the hypnotic state. J Physiol Paris. 2006;99:463–469.

[37] Frackowiak RSJ, Friston KJ, Frith CD, Dolan RJ, Mazziotta JC, editors. San Diego: Academic Press; 1997. Human brain function.

[38] Friston et al. Statistical parametric maps in functional imaging: a general linear approach. Hum Brain Mapp, 1995; 2: 173-181.

[39] Friston et al. Event-related fMRI: characterizing differential responses. Neuroimage, 1998; 7: 30-40

[40] Fransson et al. The precuneus/posterior cingulate cortex plays a pivotal role in the default mode network: Evidence from a partial correlation network analysis. Neuroimage. 2008;42:1178–1184.

[41] Gonçalves,et al. Correlating the alpha rhythm to BOLD using simultaneous EEG-fMRI: inter-subject variability. Neuroimage, 2006; 30: 203-213;

[42] Gotman et al. Combining EEG and fMRI in epilepsy: methodological challenges and clinical results. I Clin Neurophysiol, 2004; 21: 229-240

[43] Gotman et al. Generalized epileptic discharges show thalamocortical activation and the suspension of the default state of the brain. PNAS, 2005; 142: 15236-15240

[44] Gotman et al. Epileptic networks studied with EEG-fMRI. Epilepsia, 2008; 49 Suppl 3:42-51.

[45] Gusnard et al. Medial prefrontal cortex and self-referential mental activity: relation to a default mode of brain function. Proc Natl Acad Sci USA. 2001;98:4259–4264.

[46] Gusnard et al. Searching for a baseline: functional imaging and the resting human brain. Nat Rev Neurosci. 2001;2:685–694.

[47] Hamandi et al. EEG-fMRI of Generalized Spike-Wave Activity. Neuroimage. 2006;31:1700–1710.

[48] Hamandi et al. BOLD and perfusion changes during epileptic generalised spike wave activity. Neuroimage. 2008;39:608–618.

[49] Hammers et al. Abnormalities of grey and white matter [11C] flumazenil binding in temporal lobe epilepsy with normal MRI. Brain 2002; 125: 2257-2271

[50] Henry et al. Positron emission tomography. In: J. Engel, Jr. (Ed.), Surgical Treatment of Epilepsies, 2nd edn, Raven Press, New York, 1993: pp. 211-232

[51] Hill et al. Haemodynamic and metabolic aspects of photosensitive epilepsy revealled by functional magnetic resonance imaging and magnetic resonance spectroscopy. Epilepsia. 1999;40:912–920.

[52] Holmes et al. Are "generalized" seizures truly generalized? Evidence of localized mesial frontal and frontopolar discharges in absence. Epilepsia. 2004;45:1568–1579.

[53] Huggs et al. Normalization of controlateral metabolic function following temporal lobectomy demonstrated by 1H magnetic resonance spectroscopic imaging. Ann Neurol 1996; 40: 236-239

[54] Iannetti et al. fMRI/EEG in paroxysmal activity elicited by elimination of central vision and fixation. Neurology, 2002; 58: 976–979.

[55] Ives et al. Monitoring the patient's EEG during echo planar MRI. EEG and Clin Neurophysiol, 1993; 87: 417-420

[56] Kobayashi et al. Intrisic epileptogenicity in polymicrogyric cortex suggested by EEG-fMRI BOLD responses. Neurology, 2005; 64: 1263-1266

[57] Kobayashi et al. Grey matter heterotopia: what EEG-fMRI can tell us about epileptogenicity of neuronal migration disorder. Brain, 2006; 129: 366-374

[58] Kobayashi et al. Widespread and intense BOLD changes during brief focal electrographic seizures. Neurology, 2006; 66: 1049-1055

[59] Kobayashi et al. Negative BOLD responses to epileptic spikes. Human Brain Mapping, 2006; 27: 488-497

[60] Kobayashi et al.Temporal and extratemporal BOLD responses to temporal lobe interictal spikes. Epilepsia, 2006; 47: 343-354

[61] Kokkinos et al. "Epileptogenic networks in two patients with hypothalamic hamartoma." Brain Topogr. 2012;25(3):327-31.

[62] Krakow et al. EEG-fMRI of interictal epileptiform activity in patients with partial seizures. Brain, 1999; 122: 1679-1688

[63] Krakow et al. Spatio-temporal imaging of focal interictal epileptiform activity using EEG-triggered functional MRI. Epileptic Disord, 2001; 3: 67-74

[64] Kuzniecky et al.Cortical dysplasia in temporal lobe epilepsy: magnetic resonance imaging correlations. Ann. Neurol, 1991; 29: 293-298

[65] Krausz et al. Brain SPECT imaging in temporal lobe epilepsy. Neuroradiol 1991; 33: 274-276.

[66] Labate et al. Typical childhood absence seizures are associated with thalamic activation. Epileptic Disord. 2005;7:373–377.

[67] Laufs et al. EEG-fMRI mapping of asymmetrical delta activity in a patient with re-fractory epilepsy is concordant with the epileptogenic region determined by intracra-nial EEG. Magnetic Resonance Imaging, 2006/a; 24: 367-371

[68] Laufs et al. linking generalized spike-and wave discharges and resting state brain ac-tivity by using EEG-fMRI in a patient with absence seizures. Epilepsia, 2006; 47: 444-448

[69] Laufs et al. Linking Generalized Spike-and-Wave Discharges and Resting State Brain Activity by Using EEG-fMRI in a Patient with Absence Seizures. Epilepsia. 2006;47:444–448.

[70] Laufs et al. Electroencephalography/functional MRI in human epilepsy: what it cur-rently can and cannot do. Curr Opin Neurol. 2007;20:417–423.

[71] Laureys et al. Brain function in coma, vegetative state, and related disorders. Lancet Neurol. 2004;3:537–546.

[72] Lazeyras et al. Functional MRI with simultaneous EEG recording: feasibility and ap-plication to motor and visual activation. J Magn Reson Imaging, 2001; 13: 943-948

[73] Lee et al. Single Photon emission computed tomography (SPECT) brain imaging us-ing N,N,NI-trimethyl-N-(2 hydroxy-3-methyl-5-123-iodobenzyl)-1,3-propanediamine 2 HCl (HIPDM): intractable complex partial seizures. Neurology 1986; 36:1471-1477

[74] Leiderman et al. The dynamic of metabolic change following seizures ad measured by positron emission tomography with fludeoxyglucose F 18. Arch Neurol, 1994; 51: 932-936

[75] Lemieux et al. Event-related fMRI with simultaneous and continuous EEG: descrip-tion of the method and initial case report. Neuroimage, 2001; 1: 780-787

[76] Liu et al. EEG-fMRI study of the interictal epileptic activity in patients with partial epilepsy. J Neurol Sci, 2008; 268: 117-123

[77] Logothetis et al. Neurophysiological investigation of the basis of the fMRI signal. Na-ture, 2001; 412: 150-157

[78] Manganotti et al. Continuous EEG-fMRI in patients with partial epilepsy and focal interictal slow-wave discharges on EEG. Magn Res Imaging, 2008; 26: 1089-1100.

[79] Marks et al. Localization of extra-temporal epileptic foci during single photon emis-sion computed tomography. Ann Neurol 1992; 31:250-255

[80] Meeren et al. Cortical focus drives widespread corticothalamic networks during spontaneous absence seizures in rats. J Neurosci. 2002;22:1480–1495.

[81] Meeren et al. Evolving concepts on the pathophysiology of absence seizures: the cort-ical focus theory. Arch Neurol. 2005;62:371–376.

[82] Menon et al. Imaging function in the working brain with fMRI. Curr Op Neurobiol, 2001; 11:630-636.

[83] Moeller et al. EEG-fMRI: adding to standard evaluations of patients with nonlesional frontal lobe epilepsy. Neurology 2009;73:2023–30.

[84] Newton et al. SPECT in the localisation of extra-temporale and temporal seizure foci. J Neurol Neurosurg Psychiatry, 1995; 59: 26-30

[85] Ogawa et al. Brain Magnetic Resonance Imaging with contrast dependent on blood oxygenation. Proc Natl Acad Sci, 1990; 87: 9868-9872

[86] Petroff et al. GABA and glutamate in the human brain. Neuroscientist, 2002; 8: 562-573

[87] Polack et al. Deep Layer Somatosensory Cortical Neurons Initiate Spike and Wave Discharges in a Genetic Model of Absence Seizures. J Neurosci. 2007; 27:6590–6599.

[88] Prichard et al. Fuctional study of the brain by NMR. J Cereb Blood Metab, 1994; 14: 365-372

[89] Puce et al. Functional Magnetic Resonance Imaging of sensory and motor cortex: comparision with electrophysiological localisations. I Neurosurg, 1995; 83: 262-270

[90] Ruben et al. Neuroimaging of epilepsy: therapeutic implications. Neurorx, 2005; 2: 384-393

[91] Salek-Haddadi. Functional magnetic resonance imaging of human absence seizures. Ann Neurol, 2003; 53: 663-667

[92] Salek-Haddadi et al. Hemodynamic correlates of epileptiform discharges: an EEG-fMRI study of 63 patients with focal epilepsy. Brain Research, 2006; 1088: 148-166

[93] Salmenpera TM, Duncan JS. Imaging in epilepsy J. Neurol Neurosurg Psychiatry 2005;76:2–10.

[94] So. Mesial frontal epilepsy. Epilepsia, 1998; 39(Suppl 4):S49–61.

[95] Steriade et al. Spike-Wave Complexes and Fast Components of Cortically Generated Seizures. I. Role of Neocortex and Thalamus. J Neurophysiol. 1998;80:1439–1455.

[96] Tai et al. Applications of positron emission tomography (PET) in Neurology. J. Neurol Neurosurg Psych, 2004; 75: 669-676.

[97] Thorton et al. EEG correlated functional MRI and postoperative outcome in focal epilepsy. J Neurol Neurosurg Psychiatry,2010; 81:922-927.

[98] Tucker et al. Discharges in ventromedial frontal cortex during absence spells. Epilepsy Behav. 2007;11:546–557.

[99] Vaudano. Causal hierarchy within the thalamo-cortical network in spike and wave discharges. PLoS One, 2009; 4(8):e6475

[100] Westmoreland. The EEG findings in extratemporal seizures. Epilepsia, 1998; 39(Suppl 4):S1–8.

Chapter 6

Brain Function in Fibromyalgia: Altered Pain Processing and Cognitive Dysfunction

Francisco Mercado, Paloma Barjola,
Marisa Fernández-Sánchez, Virginia Guerra and
Francisco Gómez-Esquer

Additional information is available at the end of the chapter

1. Introduction

Since several decades ago chronic pain understanding has become in one of the most intriguing challenges for health professionals (rheumatologists, psychologists, physiotherapists, anaesthesiologists, pharmacologists, etc). Different reasons are behind that traditionally poor knowledge about the etiology, mechanisms and treatment of chronic pain. Pain has been very often considered as a peripheral entity in which peripheral causes, such as inflammation and structural joint damage, have been only explored. Thus, difficulties to explain painful symptomatology associated to chronic pain patients, such as the great discordance between pain complaints or severity and their supposed peripheral causes, have lead to the development of investigations to advance in the knowledge of pain mechanisms in chronic pain diseases (p.e., non-inflammatory conditions), such as it occurs in fibromyalgia (Buskila, 2009). These studies have highlighted both the important role of central pain-processing mechanisms and its evidently multifactorial status (Lee et al., 2011; Schweinhardt et al., 2008).

Fibromyalgia (FM) constitutes a chronic syndrome mainly characterized by the presence of widespread and diffuse pain (Fan, 2004). Traditionally, FM diagnosis has been only established by the presence of widespread pain during at least three months and tenderness to palpation at specific locations (the so-called 'tender points') following the American College of Rheumatology criteria (ACR, Wolfe et al., 1990). refer to 18 places symmetrically distributed at both sides of the body where patients feel pain when a weak pressure is applied on them with the thumb of the examiner (lower than 4kg/cm2, see Figure 1). Currently, this syndrome is affecting between 2-4% of population (between 80 and 90 percent of patients diagnosed with FM are women) being one of the most common causes of pain and disability. However, the biological bases for the clinical characteristics of FM remain elusive (Martínez-Lavin, 2004; Montoya et al., 2005; Vierck, 2006). Studies have focused particularly on the mechanisms underlying pain perception, and central signals processing. FM patients refer two kinds of somatic sensations: a) enhanced pain sensitivity to painful stimulation (hyperalgesia) and b) a painful response to a normally innocuous stimulus (allodynia). Central augmentation mechanisms underlying this amplified pain perception have been investigated using advanced imaging techniques that aim to localize and describe alterations in specific areas of the brain. Indeed, scientific evidence suggests that central abnormalities in the processing of pain signals seem to be responsible of such altered pain manifestations (diffuse hyperalgesia and allodynia) in FM (Staud et al., 2004; Thieme et al., 2005).

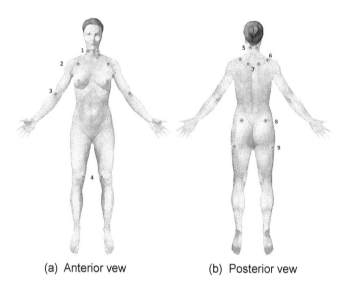

(a) Anterior vew   (b) Posterior vew

Figure 1. Bilateral tender point locations for the traditional ACR diagnosis criteria for Fibromyalgia (adapted from Wolfe et al., 1990). (a) ANTERIOR VIEW: 1. *Low cervical*: the anterior aspects of the intertransverse spaces at C5-C7, 2. *Second rib*: the second costochondral junctions, lateral to the junctions on upper surfaces, 3. *Lateral epicondyle*: 2cm distal to the epicondyles, 4. *Knee*: the medial fat pad proximal to the joint line. (b) POSTERIOR VIEW: 5. *Occiput*: the suboccipital muscle insertions, 6. *Trapezius*: the midpoint of the upper border, 7. *Supraspinatus*: above the scapula spine near the medial border, 8. *Gluteal*: upper outer quadrants of buttocks in anterior fold of muscle, 9. *Greater trochanter*: posterior to the trochanteric prominence.

Additionally, people with FM frequently experience a great amount of other accompanying symptoms apart from pain, such as physical complaints (stiffness, fatigue, sleep problems), affective disorders (anxiety or depression) and cognitive dysfunctions (failures in memory, attention and concentration). In fact, cognitive failures represent one of the most important complaints of these patients, recently denominated as *fibrofog* (Glass, 2010), leading to produce even greater functional impact than pain itself (Glass, 2009). Based on growing evidence from neuropsychological and neuroimaging studies, ACR criteria have been recently modified including the cognitive dysfunction and affective disturbances, among other symptoms, as key factors for FM diagnosis (Wolfe et al., 2010). These findings, along with the lack of peripheral signs of inflammation to account for pain, support the hypothesis that FM is a syndrome characterized by an abnormal processing of information at the level of central nervous system. Therefore, psychoneurobiologic dysfunctions seem to be crucial for trying to explain this multifactorial and still not fully understood clinical condition (Lee et al., 2011; Schweinhardt et al., 2008), but also to give response, at least partially, to the appearance and maintenance of both pain-related and cognitive symptomatology. In the following review, we will try to describe what is currently known about the cerebral mechanisms in pain processing, the neural correlates of cognitive dysfunction and the pathogenesis of FM, with special attention to the genetic basis.

2. Cerebral pain processing in fibromyalgia

Fibromyalgia is considered a chronic pain syndrome which cause (still remain elusive) does not have been found in localized lesions, inflammatory processes or damage to the joints, muscles or other tissues. Experimental evidence indicates that pain processing abnormalities leading to maintenance of pain showed by these patients (e.g., hyperalgesic states) could be due to both central sensitization mechanisms and specific defects in central pain processing related to the loss of normal activity of descending pain-inhibitory (e.g., serotonin-norephi-nephrine-opioidergic) pathways (Ceko et al., 2012; Lee et al., 2011). Central sensitization related to diffuse hyperalgesia and allodynia is functionally linked to central nervous changes caused by the release of different excitatory neurotransmitters such as serotonin, substance P or glutamate, among others. Through their action on specific receptors (e.g., NMDA) those neurotransmitters might produce enhanced and amplified responses at central nervous level (Woolf, 2004). Specifically, central sensitization can also produce an augmentation of receptive fields in neurons belonging to spinal cord and peripheral fibers. Other neurophysiological indices found in FM patients have involved elevated levels of substance P and serotonin metabolites in cerebrospinal fluid compared with healthy people (Russell et al., 1994; Russell et al., 1992), along with a diminished level of neurotransmitters, which dampen pain sensitivity response (e.g., norepinephrine) suggesting again defects in central pain processing (Russell et al., 1992). Behaviourally, the phenomenon of central sensitization is characterized by lower thresholds in pain perception, pain tolerance and by an enhancement of noxious sensations as a consequence of repeated stimulation, as it occurs in temporal summation (Staud et al., 2003). Additionally, whereas the activation of NMDA receptor channels produces central sensitization, the administration of NMDA receptor antagonists such as ketamine reduces significantly pain perception and facilitates the inhibition of hyperalgesia indices (i.e., temporal summation) in FM patients (Price et al., 2002; Graven-Nielsen et al., 2000). Neuroi-maging studies have demonstrated the presence of an augmented activation pattern of pain processing involving several cortical and subcortical regions in FM (Gracely et al., 2002). This augmented pain processing pattern resulted in response to the same perceived intensity of painful stimulation compared to control participants (Gracely et al., 2002; Cook et al., 2004).

Pain descending inhibitory pathways start from different cerebral levels localized on the brainstem, bulbar region, diencephalic structures and cortical areas. These pathways constitute one of the most important mechanisms involved in the pain perception modulation of sensory information in the dorsal horn of spinal cord. Experimental evidence has described defects in those pain inhibitory pathways leading to a loss of descending endogenous analgesia and the maintenance and enhancement of painful sensations in patients with FM (Julien et al., 2005). These results have been found using different types of acute noxious stimulation. Staud and colleagues (2003) highlighted the presence of diminished pain inhibitory mechanisms in response to hot water in a sample of women with and without FM. Previous studies applying tonic thermal stimulation and by using a tourniquet to produce ischemic pain showed evidence for the defects in descending inhibitory pain activity in FM (Lautenbacher et al., 1997; Kosek et al., 1997). In the same line, diminished periaqueductal gray responses to heat stimulation have been reported in these patients when it was compared with the activity of healthy participants (Cook et al., 2004). Periaqueductal gray region (PGR) has been described as an important structure involved in both ascending and descending pain processing signals (Stahl, 2009). Descending projections from PGR to dorsolateral pontine structures act inhibiting pain signals from peripheral afferent neurons in the dorsal horn of the spinal cord through the release of noradrenaline and serotonin neurotransmitters. Thus, the observed lack of activation within PGR in FM could lead to a loss of descending analgesia enhancing chronic responses of hyperalgesia in these patients (Herrero et al., 2000). Exposed findings demonstrate the main role of abnormalities in central mechanisms as an important key to understand chronic pain in the FM syndrome (Abeles et al., 2007; Bennett, 2005; Lee et al., 2011).

2.1. Morphological brain changes associated with abnormal pain processing in fibromyalgia

Experimental evidence focused on the study of brain areas involved in the processing of painful stimulation has revealed that chronic pain patients show an abnormal activation pattern at specified brain regions (e.g., Kwiatek et al., 2000). Neuroimaging research and its application to the study of pain, has facilitated the identification of a brain network involved in pain processing that has been denominated as 'pain matrix', comprised, among others, by different cortical and subcortical regions: for example, somatosensory regions, insular areas and anterior cingulated cortices (ACC) (Bushnell et al., 2005; Tracey &Mantyh, 2007). Although recently the referred pain matrix has been functionally redefined not only as a pain processing network but also as salience detection system (Iannetti et al., 2010; Legrain et al., 2011; Tracey & Johns, 2010), the role played by somatosensory cortices and other cortical regions, such as posterior parietal cortex or prefrontal areas in the processing of nociceptive signals and in the affective/cognitive modulation processes of pain perception, has been extensively documented (Lorenz et al., 2003; Peyron et al., 2000; Rolls et al., 2003; Sawamoto et al., 2000; Singer et al., 2004; Wiech et al., 2008). For instance, attentional modulations on pain perception have been seen in the increase and/or decrease of activations within insula and ACC (Valet et al., 2004; Wiech et al., 2005).

Chronic pain diseases are commonly characterized by an abnormal functioning when painful events are processed and as a consequence of it, chronic pain has been understood as an altered perceptual state (Apkarian et al., 2005). Nevertheless, chronic pain is also defined as a dysfunctional condition derived from the appearance of structural brain changes that become more generalized as a function of the years suffering from pain (Baliki et al., 2011). Such changes could cause a dysfunctional neural reorganization affecting brain dynamics (Baliki et al., 2008; Tagliazucchi et al., 2010). Evidence accumulated from the last years through the use of different brain imaging methodologies supports the presence of changes in the brain of FM patients (i.e., structural and functional changes) (García-Campayo et al., 2010; Gracely et al., 2011), although such changes are heterogeneous and a unique interpretation about its clinical meaning remains still unclear. Altered brain morphology was reported by voxel-based morphometry (VBM) studies showing that FM patients had less grey matter density than healthy subjects in several brain regions including insula and ACC (Kuchinad et al., 2007). However, grey matter increase in other cerebral areas belonging to the somatosensory system, such as the Striatum or in those other ones involved in the cognitive modulation of pain (i.e., Orbitofrontal Cortex-OFC) have been seen in patients suffering from FM (Schmidt-Wilcke et al., 2007). Further findings combining diffusion-tensor imaging (DTI) and VBM methodologies have described not only a reduction in grey matter density in FM but also abnormalities in white matter microstructure within thalamus and insular cortex, being highly correlated with the intensity of main FM symptoms (Lutz et al., 2008). Specifically, patients showing higher pain intensity scores were characterized by DTI measurements indicating changes within superior frontal gyrus (SFG). Moreover, changes in SFG and ACC were positively correlated with increased fatigue and self-perceived physical impairment. Affective symptoms defined by higher scores in posttraumatic stress scales were negatively correlated with microstructural changes represented by values of fractional anisotropy (FA) in FM. In this line, Hsu and colleagues (2009) reported decreased grey matter volume in the left anterior insula for patients with FM compared to healthy control participants. This difference in grey matter volume disappeared when the presence of affective disorders in FM patients was controlled. Thus, grey matter volume within this area was inversely correlated with scores in trait anxiety, highlighting the important role of affective disturbances in the explanation of these morphological brain changes. More recent studies have documented that patients with FM syndrome show grey matter atrophy within ACC, mid-cingulate Cortex (MCC) and insular cortex, but affective symptoms like depression are not related to these grey matter changes (Robinson et al., 2011). Along with emotional symptomatology, cognitive alterations in FM have been correlated with changes in grey matter values (Luerding et al., 2008). They found that working memory performance in FM patients was highly and positively correlated with decreased grey matter values within medial prefrontal cortex (MPFC) and ACC, showing that cognitive deficits in FM are associated with changes in brain morphology.

Therefore, mentioned brain abnormalities in the traditionally denominated pain matrix regions might contribute to the alteration of pain processing in FM patients, but they could also affect other domains such as cognitive and affective symptomatology. In fact, it has been proposed that pain and cognitive impairment in FM may co-occur sharing underlying neural networks (Luerding et al., 2008), and as a consequence of it, performance derived from carrying out a cognitive task when individual is in pain might decrease due to the availability of neural resources is limited and they are invested in pain processing (Seminowicz and Davis, 2007). Additionally, the presence of chronic pain along the years might contribute to the appearance of changes in the brain leading to abnormal activation of brain regions that could exacerbate pain itself and also disturb cognitive function in FM (Kuchinad et al., 2007). Although structural neuroimaging evidence supports the association of chronic pain in FM with grey matter abnormalities, future investigations should be projected to confirm and extend these findings.

2.2. Functional brain changes associated with abnormal pain processing in fibromyalgia

Beyond morphological brain changes, functional imaging investigations have revealed abnormal activation patterns at specific cerebral regions in FM patients (e.g., Cook et al., 2004), however, these anomalies in pain processing are not always circumscribed to activation of brain areas intimately or traditionally related to pain. It has been observed during different experimental situations: in response to painful stimulation, when somatosensory (not painful) information has to be processed and even during resting-state conditions. One of the first neuroimaging studies conducted to investigate such issues demonstrated enhanced brain activation in many regions (i.e., primary and secondary somatosensory cortex, ACC, insula) for FM patients in response to similar levels of pressure stimulation to that one applied to control subjects (Gracely et al., 2002). Moreover, when subjectively painful conditions were established to be comparable (i.e., intensity of stimulation was significantly greater to healthy people than patients for provoke a similar subjective level of pain perception) similar brain activation patterns were found between both patients and control groups. These results indicate that central sensitization defects could be explaining the presence of such augmented activation pattern for painful signals in FM. More recent studies aimed to test the hypothesis of central augmentation pain processing in FM have confirmed and extended those findings (Maestú et al., 2013). Abnormal brain activation of different regions related to the affective/ motivational components of pain processing was found in patients with FM during a pain situation induced by a small incision into the skin (Burgmer et al., 2009). Thus, enhanced activations were observed within frontal and cingulated cortices, along with supplementary motor areas. Such altered responses were especially prominent during the pain anticipation period. Additionally, that altered temporal BOLD-signal pattern was found as specific for FM patients when they were compared to other patients suffering from rheumatoid arthritis (Burgmer et al., 2010). It leads to think that fronto-cingulated regions could play a key role as central mechanisms of pain processing responsible to the maintenance and exacerbation of chronic pain in FM.

Previous investigations had already given data about the role of cognitive, affective and social factors on pain processing in FM. Neural responses to somatosensory stimuli can be modulated by cognitive and emotional factors (Cook et al., 2004). Specifically, the catastrophyzing thinking style has been associated with enhanced cerebral responses to pain. Cortical areas involved in pain expectancy or pain-related attention (ACC, MPFC or dorsolateral prefrontal cortex –DLPFC-) showed more intense activity in FM patients who scored high in catastrophizing (Gracely et al., 2004). Affective conditions such as comorbid depression, seem to have influence in the activation of amygdala, but not of somatosensory brain regions during pain processing information (Giesecke et al., 2005). Event-related potentials (ERP) studies have also provided data demonstrating abnormal emotional modulation of brain processing in response to somatosensory/non-painful stimuli (Montoya et al., 2005). Somatosensory components (i.e, P50) displayed largest amplitudes when FM patients were introduced within a negative emotional context created with unpleasant slides. The influence of the emotional context was also described during the processing of painful stimulation (Montoya et al., 2004). At the same time, the presence of significant others during the application of painful stimulation was found as a social factor that diminish magnetic brain responses and subjective pain in FM patients compared to control participants (Montoya et al., 2004). Other works have observed that FM patients show a significant enhancement of brain activation within regions involved in the emotional/cognitive aspects linked to pain processing as compared to control subjects, given a painful stimulation (Burgmer et al., 2009). Indeed, larger activation within CCA and anterior insula along with more persisting responses in insular cortex were found for FM patients as well (Pujol et al., 2009). It supports the hypothesis that both affective/cognitive and social factors may play a very important role for pain processing in patients with FM.

On the other hand, the role played by several neurotransmitters, such as dopamine or glutamate, which exerts their functions at the level of central neural system, has been also highlighted in the pathogenesis of FM and studied through the use of neuroimaging techniques (Harris, 2010; Stahl, 2009). Different genetic polymorphisms associated with the functional activity of those neuromodulators have been documented (Ablin et al., 2008), as it will be extensively described later. Evidence on altered levels of mentioned neurotransmitters within the brain of patients with FM has recently reported (Harris et al., 2008; 2009). Dysregulation in levels of glutamate, an excitatory neurotransmitter, has been found within the posterior insula of FM patients being such altered levels associated with experimental pain (Harris et al., 2010). Higher concentration levels of glutamate and glutamine were also detected within the amygdala (Valdés et al., 2010) and posterior insula (Fayed et al., 2010). Patients group showed diminished pain thresholds and high scores in pain and tenderness suggesting that neuronal hiperexcitability elicited by the presence of glutamate may lead to an augmented central pain processing. With respect to other neurotransmitters, different investigations have indicated an abnormal dopamine response to pain in FM (Wood et al., 2007b; Wood et al., 2009). It is known that dopamine is a neurotransmitter involved in pain modulation, but whereas general population showed an increase of dopamine release when a painful stimulus was perceived FM patients did not (Wood et al., 2007a). Thus, that deficiency in dopaminergic reactivity might have a relevant impact on the development and maintenance of chronic pain in FM. In fact, some studies have shown reduced presynaptic dopaminergic activity suggesting that such disrupted neurotransmission could prevent for natural analgesia in FM (Wood et al., 2007b). More recent findings have associated alterations in dopaminergic neurotransmission with a decrease in grey matter density within posterior cingulated cortex, ACC and parahippocampal gyri (Wood et al., 2009). Therefore, these data suggest that pharmacological approaches targeted to the specific or combined use of glutamatergic and dopaminergic treatments may be effective and should be explored (for a review see, Smith-Wilcke & Clauw, 2010).

Finally, recent investigations postulate that FM could be characterized by an alteration of brain connectivity among different brain networks (Cifre et al., 2012; Napadow et al., 2010). It has been documented that chronic pain produces a disruption in the default mode network (DMN;

Baliki et al., 2008). Evidence coming from neuroimaging studies reported increased resting state connectivity between insula and other brain networks such as the DMN in FM patients. This connectivity pattern was highly and positively correlated with spontaneous pain (Napadow et al., 2010). In fact, when a sample of patients underwent to an acupuncture treatment aimed to diminish pain perception, the degree of connectivity between insula and DMN was also decreased leading to consider resting state connectivity as an objective marker to assess pain in FM (Napadow et al., 2012). Other studies have confirmed the presence of an altered connectivity pattern among brain regions belonging to pain processing network in FM during rest (Cifre et al., 2012). Indeed, such alteration might be due to slow temporal summation effects evoked by C-fiber pain (Craggs et al., 2012).

3. Neural correlates of cognitive dysfunction in fibromyalgia

3.1. Cognitive complaints in FM

It has been suggested that FM syndrome is characterized by an abnormal processing of information in the central nervous system (Montoya et al., 2005; Okijufi et al., 2002) affecting the response to somatosensory stimulation (e.g., painful signals) but also to information belonging to other modalities (e.g., visual, auditory, etc). Several studies indicate that apart from pain and other physical symptoms, cognitive failures are referred by these patients as one of the most important complaints (recently denominated as *fibrofog*; Glass, 2009; Williams et al., 2011), leading to produce even greater functional impact than pain itself (Arnold et al., 2008; Glass et al., 2005). Thus, the incidence rate for memory and concentration difficulties exceeds 90% in FM, being significantly higher that one occurred in other chronic pain conditions (Arnold et al., 2008; Mease et al., 2008). Additionally, self-reports of patients support the presence of a higher number of cognitive problems than patients suffering from other chronic pain syndromes (Katz et al., 2004), affecting several cognitive domains (Williams et al., 2011). For example, memory complaints of FM patients were positively correlated with the objective perfomance obtained in tasks which set in motion memory resources (Glass et al., 2005). Moreover, these cognitive difficulties manifest persistently in many of daily activities involving the allocation of attentional control resources such as to remember that they have to call someone the next day or to inhibit thoughts that do not allow them to develop other concurrent daily tasks. Experimental evidence confirms that attention, concentration, episodic memory and verbal fluency are impaired in FM (Glass, 2009) showing that such difficulties in the processing of information constitute a very disruptive symptom for patients who have FM, worsening its quality of life and leading to consider it as an independent symptom (Schmidt-Wilcke *et al.*, 2010).

3.2. Neuropsychological and behavioural data on cognitive dysfunction in FM

Since the beginning of the past decade growing objective evidence based mainly on neuropsychological studies has shown real and significant impairments of cognitive functions in FM (Glass & Park, 2001; Park et al., 2001). First attempts to characterize dyscognition in FM reported deficits in the two declarative memory systems related to the explicit recall of information, episodic and semantic memory. Experimental data revealed poor performance on both standardized (Grace et al., 1999) and non-standarized episodic memory tests (Landro et al., 1997; Grisart et al., 2002). Semantic memory problems have also been documented. FM group showed lower ability for accessing to stored general knowledge than control group when patients were asked to report as many words as they could say starting with a given letter (for example, 'p') and belonging to a specific category (for example, 'fruits and vegetables') (Landro et al., 1997; Park et al., 2001). Along with verbal fluency difficulties, a decrease in naming speed (Leavitt et al., 2008) and speed processing (Veldhuijzen et al., 2012) was also found in FM patients. However, those results are not unequivocal since some studies failed to find differences in cognitive function between patients and healthy control participants (Suhr, 2003). This variability could be related to the lack of previous systematic and detailed research, suggesting that cognitive impairment in FM patients is not generalized; rather is specific-process dependent.

Recent data have suggested that findings on cognitive dysfunction in FM are particularly solid when patients have to deal with tasks demanding for both executive control and working memory resources (Ambrose et al., 2012; Glass, 2010). Impairments in those domains seem to be the key to explain a great part of the cognitive dysfunction in FM. Executive functions (EF) refer to those mechanisms that allow the regulation of both behaviour and other cognitive processes to achieve a specific objective (Muñoz-Céspedes and Tirapu, 2001). Within this theoretical frame, working memory is defined as the support system of those EF aimed to temporarily hold in mind and manage with a variable amount of information (Baddeley, 2000). Thus, working memory dysfunctions have also been seen in FM (Luerding et al., 2008). It has been also observed that patients perform poorly in a variety of tasks involving the allocation of executive control resources to alternate between cognitive sets (Verdejo-García et al., 2009) and to make emotional decisions (Verdejo-García et al., 2009; Walteros et al., 2011) or to face with a task-switching test (Glass, 2006). Tests commonly used to study those executive function processes are Wisconsin Card Sorting Test (WCST) and the Iowa Gambling Task (IGT). Several studies using the Paced Auditory Serial Attention Test (PASAT) have detected a diminished perfomance in FM individuals compared to controls (Leavitt & Katz, 2006; Munguía-Izquierdo et al., 2008). Other working memory components like response inhibition are also suggested to be impaired in FM (Correa et al., 2011). Very similar results have been found during the performance in those tests with a high degree of ecological validity (Test of Everyday Attention, TEA) that includes everyday attentional tasks (Dick et al., 2008). Working memory components measured by TEA were impaired in FM, especially when stimuli competition had to be solved. In this sense, the fact that attentional control difficulties become more evident during distraction (derived from a situation of stimuli competition) has lead to consider it as a key point to better understand cognitive dysfunction in FM (Leavitt & Katz, 2006). It was proposed that failures to inhibit competing stimulation might be an explanation for this difficulty; due to FM patients show hypersensitivity to process information coming from any sensorial modality (Geisser et al., 2008). Such general distractibility could be translated into an attentional orientation towards any type of task-irrelevant stimuli (González et al., 2010) leading to difficulties to focalize attention on relevant information. However, recent data derived from the use of cognitive inhibition tests indicate that patients with FM do not show a specific problem in such processes (Veldhuijzen et al., 2012).

Although the body of research on cognitive dysfunction in FM has strongly grown in recent years, there are still several unexplored issues in this field of knowledge that should be investigated such as the delimitation of the specific cognitive mechanisms that are altered in these patients. For instance, it is accepted that working memory abilities are impaired in FM, but are different components (e.g., temporal holding of information, inhibition, manage with two concurrent tasks, etc) characterizing working memory equally affected? Kim and colleagues (2012) have indicated that memory is selectively impaired in FM showing the possible existence of a memory dissociation. Data coming from neuropsychological assessments reveal that whereas visuospatial memory abilities are dysfunctional, verbal memory is quite unaffected. Following a similar reasoning, several studies postulate that cognitive dysfunction in FM is restricted to those cognitive mechanisms based on controlled processes (Grisart et al., 2002). However, the presence of a generalized hypervigilance response in FM (Carrillo de la Peña et al., 2006) seems to be under the control of automatic processes, rather than controlled ones (Crombez et al., 2005). Moreover, recent data have demonstrated a reduced performance of patients with FM during an implicit memory task (Duschek et al., 2013). It is the first direct evidence of cognitive disruption associated with processes non-dependent from conscious and controlled resources in FM. Finally, several comorbid symptoms of FM (e.g., anxiety, depression, sleep disturbances, medication, pain, etc) have been associated with a worsening of cognitive dysfunction. Although the impact of affective symptomatology (anxiety and depression) and sleep problems on the cognitive dysfunction in FM might be important, these variables do not entirely explain it (Park et al., 2001; Dick et al., 2008). However, the negative impact of both chronic and acute pain seems to be very robust. When this variable is controlled FM patients show a marked impairment in tasks involving different cognitive domains (Glass et al., 2011; Reyes del Paso et al., 2012; Verdejo-García et al., 2009). Additionally, level of self-reported pain is correlated with cognitive performance in FM (Glass et al., 2005) and it has been highlighted as a mediating variable to explain deficits in self-regulatory processes in these patients (Solberg et al., 2010). Therefore, the role of pain on cognitive disturbances is considered as quite relevant. Nevertheless, the neurocognitive mechanisms by means pain interferes on patient's cognitive function are still unknown.

3.3. Brain activity related to cognitive dysfunction in FM

As it was previously indicated, accumulated evidence supports the presence of clear objective impairments in cognitive function of patients with FM. Cognitive dysfunctional pattern associated with FM (i.e., executive control deficits, working memory failures and declarative memory difficulties) points out to the existence of an altered neural substrate, presumably at least within prefrontal regions, such as inferior prefrontal cortex (IPC), MPFC or ACC along with their connexions with temporal and parietal regions (Glass, 2010; Glass et al., 2011). Although studies focused on these neural mechanisms underlying dysfunctional cognitive processes in FM are still surprisingly scarce, new findings cast some light on the possible altered neurocognitive mechanisms. In this sense, neuroimaging investigations have repeatedly showed increased haemodynamic activity at prefrontal regions (i.e., dorsolateral pre-frontal cortex –DLPFC-, ventromedial prefrontal –VMPFC- cortex and ACC) during tasks involving working memory and executive control processes (Bunge et al., 2000; Dagher et al., 1999). Moreover, Altamura and coworkers (2007) have highlighted that the right allocation of working memory resources to accomplish a given task depends on prefrontal regions.

Specific data related to FM patients, have found that working memory performance in FM patients was highly and positively correlated with grey matter values within MPFC and ACC, showing that a decrease of grey matter volume within those prefrontal regions is associated with working memory deficits in FM (Luerding et al., 2008). Additionally, recent functional neuroimaging investigations have revealed diminished activations in cortical regions belong-ing to the inhibition network, such as ACC, mid-cingulated cortex (MCC) and motor process-ing areas in patients with FM during the performance in a simple go/no-go task (Glass et al., 2011). At the same time, inefficient activations were detected within insular cortex and IFG when patients had to perform on the mentioned response motor inhibition task. It has been suggested that such effects might be explained via either a greater brain recruitment of cortical compensatory regions different from those involved in response inhibition network. Extend-ing such findings, our research group has tried to characterize cognitive inhibition mecha-nisms, as part of the altered working memory functions, in patients with FM. Patients showed both enhanced P450 amplitudes and brain activations within IFG in response to an emotional Stroop task (Mercado et al., in press). More in detail, symptom-related words were the kind of stimulation that elicited both the greater frontal P450 amplitudes and the higher IFG activations as compared to rest of stimuli (i.e., general negative-arousing, positive-arousing and neutral words; see Figures 2 and 3). This abnormally enhanced brain activity suggests the presence of a specific difficulty in cognitive inhibition in FM patients (under conditions intimately linked with the core concerns of their disease). However, such supplementary recruitment of neural resources by means same cortical areas only allow them to achieve a comparable behavioural performance to healthy control group during the cognitive inhibition task. These results are in contradiction with those coming from behavioural studies indicating intact cognitive inhibition abilities in FM (Veldhuijzen et al., 2012). A tentative explanation could be related to the idea that brain activity techniques might be more sensitive to detect subtle dysfunctions than behavioural measures alone such as often occurs in FM patients (Glass et al., 2011). Other functional neuroimaging studies have showed that working memory dysfunction (measured through a n-back task) in FM are related to a reduction of neural activity not only at prefrontal regions but also within inferior parietal cortex (IPC) (Seo et al., 2012). It suggests that a different neural activation pattern of the frontoparietal memory network could be explaining, at least partially, cognitive impairments in FM. Diminished early ERP activity of FM patients during a 2-back task has been also detected at inferior parietal sites, Suggesting that problems associated with the early storage of information might be attribut-able to analtered functioning of parietal areas (Mercado et al.,in preparation). On the other hand, some investigations have indicated the presence of differences associated with the hippocampus activity between patients and healthy control participants (Emad et al., 2008).

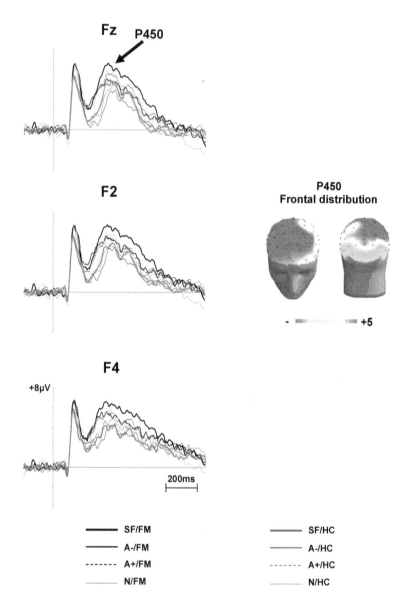

Figure 2. Grand averages of P450 component corresponding to Fibromyalgia (FM) and Healthy control (HC) participants in response to FM symptoms (SF), negative-arousing (A-), positive-arousing (A+) and neutral (N) stimuli. Scales
and polarity are shown at F4. 3D maps show topographical distribution of the P450 component. Red areas reflect high
activity.

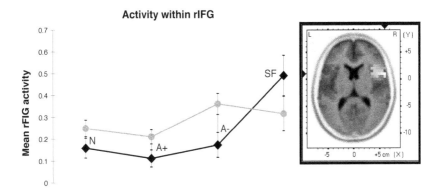

Figure 3. rIFG activity from the emotional Stroop task for patients with fibromyalgia (FM) and healthy control participants (HC). Right side shows sLORETA solutions to non-parametric randomization tests on P450 component. Coronal brain view in MNI305 template, sliced through the region of maximum activity, is illustrated. Left side shows mean rIFG activity for FM patients and HC participants across the four word categories: FM symptoms (SF), negative-arousing (A-), positive-arousing (A+) and neutral (N) stimuli. Error bars reflect standard errors. Black line represent rIFG activity for FM patients and, grey line, for HC participants.

As mentioned before, cognitive dysfunctions and pain processing may rely on partially overlapping regions in FM patients. As a consequence of this, resources taken up by pain processing may not be available for executive functioning (Glass et al., 2011). Pain level of patients might contribute to this effect over cognition. Neuroimaging techiques represent an opportunity to advance in the comprehension of FM and further studies should be done to delimitate deficits in order to develop better diagnostic and classification criteria of FM patients and to better design neuropsychological interventions oriented to increase their quality of life.

4. Genetics in fibromyalgia: Pain and cognition

Genetic predisposition is likely to be an important factor in the development of FM as suggested by several familial studies (Buskila et al., 1996, 2007; Arnold et al., 2004). These studies found that first-degree relatives of patients with FM had lower pain threshold than controls and were 8.5 times more likely to develop FM than relatives of patients with rheumatoid arthritis. The studies also indicated that the relatives of FM patients are more likely to suffer from comorbidities commonly seen in FM, such as mood disorders, irritable bowel syndrome (IBS), temporomandibular disorder (TMD) and headache (Ablin et al., 2008; Buskila et al., 1996, 2007). Identifying the genes responsible for this genetic contribution to risk should provide a better understanding of the complex mechanisms underlying FM and other chronic pain diseases. In recent years, attempts have been made to identify the genes involved in FM using candidate gene genetic association studies, which look for differences in the frequency of different polymorphisms between cases and controls, or with a quantifiable trait. The majority of such candidates have been genes involved in catecholaminergic or serotonergic neurotransmission, including receptors and transporters for dopamine, serotonin, norepinephrine, and epinephrine, as well as the catabolic enzymes catechol-O-methyltransferase (COMT).

Next we will review, in outline, the main findings made on genes associated with FM. The most widely studied gene to date is **Catechol-O-Methyltransferase (COMT)**, which degrades catecholamines such as dopamine, noradrenaline and adrenalin that are involved in various physiological functions including mood, cognition and stress response (Belfer and Segal, 2011). In particular, a single nucleotide polymorphism (SNP), (rs4680), has received a great deal of attention due its functional implications (Zubieta et al., 2003). This polymorphism causes a substitution from a valina (Val) to a methionine (Met) at amino acid position 158 (*Val158Met*), leading to a three to four fold reduced activity of the COMT enzyme (Lotta et al., 1995). In 2005, Diatchenko and colleagues described three very common haplotypes consisting of four SNPs (rs6269, rs 4633, rs4818 and rs4680-*Val158Met*) accounting for 96% of all haplotypes observed in human populations (Diatchenko et al., 2005). They identified them as low (LPS), average (APS) and high (HPS) pain sensitivity haplotypes, and they found a correlation with much more profound change in COMT activity (up to 20-fold difference).

The *met/met* genotype of the COMT *Val158Met* polymorphism has been associated with higher sensitivity in response to pain stimuli and the number of tender points in FM (Cohen et al., 2009) as well as with a high risk for the development of FM (García-Fructuoso et al., 2006; Barbosa et al., 2012). Recently, Martínez-Jauand and colleagues (2013) have shown that the HPS-APS haplotypes are more frequent in FM patients than in healthy controls and that FM patients who possess those genetic combinations displayed an increased sensitivity to experimental pain. These results are in accordance with previous reports showing a strong association between the HPS haplotype and high score on the Fibromyalgia Impact Questionnaire (Vargas-Alarcón et al., 2007). These haplotypes might be associated with increased risk of developing chronic pain disorders (Diatchenko et al., 2005). These data suggest that a decrease of COMT activity might contribute to the maintenance of pain symptoms in FM, and might play a significant role in classifying FM patients (Martínez-Jauand et al., 2013).

COMT variants moderate not only pain but also maladaptive coping processes in patients with FM. Finan and colleagues (2010 and 2011) demonstrated that Met158 allele homozygotes experience more pain in days when pain catastrophizing and pain attention scores were elevated, and a greater decline in positive affect on days when pain was elevated. These findings support the role of COMT and catecholamines in affective reactivity to pain, and in pain-related cognition pathways in patients with FM. A recent study has proposed that the Val158Met can play a relevant role in phenotypic expression of FM. They showed that women with FM and Met/Met genotype had more severe psychological and functional impact scores than those with the Val/Val genotype, although the differences were not significant (Desmeules et al., 2012). More recently, Fernández de las Peñas and colleagues (2012) have shown that FM patients with Met/Met genotype exhibit higher disability, anxiety and depression than those with Val/Val and Val/Met genotype.

As indicated above, cognitive dysfunction has been considered as one of the most disturbing symptoms, apart from pain, in patients with FM. Neuropsychological investigations have suggested that executive control and working memory impairments seem to be the key to explain a great part of this cognitive dysfunction in FM (Glass, 2010) and it points out to the existence of an altered neural substrate, presumably within prefrontal regions, such as inferior prefrontal cortex (IPFC), MPFC or ACC (Glass et al., 2011). In this context, it has been shown that more than 60% of released dopamine is metabolized by COMT in the frontal cortex (Karoum et al., 1994), and that the Val158Met polymorphism affects working memory and executive functions in healthy population (Bruder et al., 2005) and some mental disorders such as schizophrenia (Diaz-Asper et al., 2006; Hosak, 2007). Therefore, COMT may be a good candidate for the study of cognitive impairment in patients with FM.

The **endogenous serotonergic system** is comprised of the neurotransmitter serotonin (5-HT), multiple serotonin receptors (5-HT2A, 5-HT3A, 5-HT3B) and the serotonin transporter (5-HTT). This system is a key contributor to both depression and pain in FM. In fact, serotonin is decreased in FM, and selective serotonin reuptake inhibitors have some efficacy in FM (Gupta and Silman, 2004). Despite the complexity of the serotonergic pathway, research has mainly focused on a limited number of genes. Offenbaecher and colleagues (1999) analyzed the genotypes of the promoter region of the serotonin transporter gene (5-HTT) in patients with FM and healthy controls. A significantly higher frequency of the S/S genotype of the serotonin transporter promoter region was found in FM as compared to healthy participants. The S/S subgroup exhibited higher mean levels of depression and psychological distress. It was suggested that these results support the notion of an altered serotonin metabolism in at least a subgroup of patients with FM (Buskila et al., 2007). These findings were subsequently confirmed by a study analyzing Palestinian Arabs and Israeli Jews (Cohen et al., 2002). However, the study in other candidate genes within the serotonergic system failed to demonstrate a significant difference in the frequency of the polymorphism among FM patients and controls (Bondy et al., 1999; Frank et al., 2004; Matsuda et al., 2010).

The **dopaminergic system** has also been the target of extensive study in search of the genetic factors related to FM. Dopamine is a crucial neurotransmitter involved in multiple activities including pain transmission and endogenous analgesia (Wood, 2008). A single nucleotide polymorphism (Ser9Gly) in the dopamine-D3 receptor gene predicts changes in pain threshold in FM patients but not in healthy subjects (Potvin et al., 2009). In the FM group, the Ser9Gly polymorphism was a predictor of decreased thermal pain threshold and diffuse noxious inhibitory control (DNIC) efficacy (Potvin et al., 2009). Polymorphisms in the dopamine receptor 4 (DRD4) gene has also been associated with FM. Buskila and colleagues (2004) reported a significant decrease in the frequency of the 7 repeated allele in exon III of the D4 receptor gene in FM patients, who also demonstrated an association between this polymorphism and the low novelty seeking personality trait. This was considered consistent with the personality profile of FM patients, who scored high on anxiety related personality traits and low on novelty or sensation seeking. In a study of 384 subjects with DRD4 polymorphism, allele 4 was the most common, occurring in 279 of the 384 subjects (Treister et al., 2009). However, there was no change in cold tolerance, cold perception, cold pain threshold, or heat pain intensity in those subjects compared to subjects with allele 2 or allele 7 (Treister et al., 2009). Dopamine D2 receptor (DRD2) is implicated in different cognitive processes and brain disorder, and polymorphisms in this gene affect gene expression, splicing, and neuronal activity during working memory (Zhang et al., 2007). This has been demonstrated in patients with schizophrenia, whose presence relatively increased density of DRD2 (Laruelle, 1998). Curiously, it has also been observed an increased sensitivity or density of dopamine D2 receptors (DRD2) in FM patients (Malt et al., 2003). Preliminary results in our research group found a significant relationship between promoter SNP (rs12364283) in DRD2 and working memory functioning in FM patients. Specifically, we found significant differences during the performance in both Spatial Span (forward sequence) and n-back tasks. Heterozygotes (TC)-FM patients had a lower performance compared to TC-HC in both Spatial Span and n-back tasks. They also perform worse than homozygotes TT-FM patients but only in the Spatial Span task (Gómez-Esquer et al., 2012). Our results suggest that DRD2 could be playing an important role in working memory functioning in FM patients and support the implication of dopaminergic pathways in the cognitive symptoms of FM.

Another candidate gene is the β_2-adrenergic receptor (ADRB2). It mediates physiologic responses such as vasodilation and bronchial smooth-muscle relaxation, and represents a connection between the sympathetic nervous system and the immune system (Small et al., 2003; Catapano & Mangi, 2007). Alterations in the ADRB2 function have been implicated in several psychiatric and psychological disorders, including those associated with chronic pain (Lee et al., 2012). Vargas-Alarcón and colleagues (2009) reported that having the AC haplotype of the two SNPs (rs1042713 and rs1042714) was associated with an increased risk for suffering FM among Mexican and Spanish individuals. Recently, it has been published the first study to demonstrate ADRB2 polymorphism-related differences in intracellular cyclic Adenosine Monophosphate (cAMP) levels in FM Peripheral Blood Mononuclear Cells (PBMC), before and after ADRB2 stimulation. These findings suggest that ADRB2 polymorphisms may influence the response to a variety of β-adrenergic ligands and may help to explain some differences in responsiveness of FM subgroups to the adrenergic agonist medication currently approved for FM treatment (Xiao et al., 2011).

Finally, we will briefly discuss about SCN9A, a gene that encodes sodium channel in dorsal root ganglia (DRG). A consistent line of investigation suggests that autonomic nervous system dysfunction may explain the multi-system features of FM. In this context, DRG play a key role in pain perception and sodium channels located in DRG act as molecular gatekeepers of pain detection at peripheral nociceptors. Mutations in this gene have caused severe pain disorders and congenital insensitivity to pain in families, thus demonstrating a critical role in pain processing (Drenth and Waxman, 2007). In FM, Vargas Alarcón and colleagues (2012) demonstrated that, in Mexican women, the frequency of rs6754031 polymorphism of SCN9A was significantly different between FM patients and healthy controls. Interestingly, patients with

GG genotype had higher Fibromyalgia Impact Questionnaire (FIQ) scores than patients with the GT or TT genotype. These results show that there is an association between the rs6754031 polymorphism and the risk of developing FM as well as the FIQ score. This association raises the possibility that some patients with severe FM may have a DRG sodium channelopathy (Vargas-Alarcón et al., 2012). However, further investigation will be necessary in other ethnic groups with a large sample size to verify this observation.

Despite the large number of studies examining the potential contribution of the candidate gene polymorphism to FM susceptibility, many studies have produced conflicting results (Potvin et al., 2010; Frank et al., 2004; Gursoy, 2002). The explanation for these results could be that individual studies based on small sample sizes have insufficient power to detect positive associations and they are incapable of demonstrating the absence of such association. Recently, Lee and colleagues (2012) have conducted a systematic meta-analysis of seventeen candidate genes and over 35 polymorphisms were identified in studies on FM susceptibility. This meta-analysis demonstrates that the 5-HT2A receptor 102T/C polymorphism confers susceptibility to FM. In contrast, no association was found between the 5-HTTLPR S/L allele, COMT Val158Met, and susceptibility to FM. However, the authors were aware of the limitations of their meta-analysis since both the number of the studies and the number of the subjects included in such studies were too small. This may have not enough power to explore the association between the candidate gene polymorphism and FM. They could not perform the ethnic-specific meta-analysis to detect associations in ethnic groups due to limited data. They have not been able either to examine whether the candidate gene polymorphisms are associated with clinical features of FM (Lee et al., 2012). Therefore, additional research including large numbers of patients and controls is required to conclude the association of the candidate gene polymorphisms with FM. Another approach being made lately to identify genetic factors involved in FM is the use of a large-scale candidate gene approach (Smith et al., 2012). This is the largest candidate genes association study of the FM to date, analyzing 3,295 SNPs corresponding to > 350 genes involved in the biological pathways relevant to nociception, inflammation, and mood. This work observed significant differences in allele frequencies between cases and controls for several novel genes: GABRB3 (in the promoter region of the GABA-A β receptor gene), TAAR1 (trace amine-associated receptor 1), GBP1 (guanylate binding protein 1), RGS4 (regulator of G-protein signaling 4), CNR1 (CB-1 cannabinoid receptor gene), and GRIA4 (AMPA ionotropic glutamate receptor 4 subunit). Three of these genes, TAAR1, RGS4, and CNRI play roles in the modulation of analgesic pathways (Smith et al., 2012). Variation in these 4 replicated genes may serve as a basis for the development of new diagnostic approaches, and the products of these genes may contribute to the pathophysiology of FM and represent potential target for therapeutic actions.

5. Conclusions and future directions

Evidence from FM investigations indicates that psychoneurobiological dysfunctions play a relevant role in the pathophysiology of this multifactorial and still not fully understood syndrome. Specifically, it was suggested that abnormalities in central brain mechanisms are crucial in the understanding of chronic pain in FM, having little relevance the involvement of peripheral processing systems. Mechanisms of central sensitization and those involving descending inhibitory pathways, along with abnormalities in neurotransmission regulatory processes, seem to underlie patient's manifestations of hyperalgesia and allodynia, among other pain-related symptoms. Experimental findings also have demonstrated that both morphological and functional brain changes are related to widespread and diffuse pain and cognitive symptoms suffered by patients with FM.

On the other hand, patients with FM are characterized by the presence of difficulties in the processing of information reporting that it constitutes a very disruptive symptom in their everyday functioning. Cognitive disturbances are mainly related to both executive functions and working memory processes. Neuroimaging investigations have found abnormal activity within prefrontal and parietal regions when patients had to face a demanding task of executive control resources. However, many researchers are trying to answer an important question in order to advance in the knowledge on FM. Can cognitive dysfunction in FM be considered as a primary symptom like abnormal pain perception or, by contrast, is it a direct consequence of the structural or functional changes produced by pain? Based on present findings, cognitive dysfunctions and pain processing seem to share brain networks (prefrontal, supplementary motor regions and parietal cortices) and as a consequence of this, resources taken up by pain processing may not be available for executive functioning. Thus, performance in those tasks, which need a recruitment of working memory resources from the frontoparietal brain network to be correctly completed, would be very poor in FM. Neuroimaging techniques represent an opportunity to advance in the comprehension of pain and cognition interactions in FM and further studies should be done to explore such deficits and their interrelations.

Current data support the statement that FM constitutes a real syndrome characterized by the existence of multiple changes into the brain. Future investigations should be projected to extend these findings and to establish comprehensive explanations about: 1) cerebral mechanisms that provoke those changes, 2) its consequences on the functional state of patients and, 3) if brain changes constitute a reversible or permanent condition in the brain of FM patients. In this sense, different therapeutic approaches targeted to reverse such changes in the brain (e.g., pharmacological treatments, neuropsychological interventions, transcraneal magnetic stimulation, etc) may be effective and should be explored. The investigation about different genetic polymorphisms is a promising approach that may also help to improve the comprehension of the pathogenesis of this multifactorial and intriguing syndrome.

Acknowledgements

This work was supported by the grants URJC-CM-2007-1636 from the Universidad Rey Juan Carlos/ComunidadAutónoma de Madrid and PSI2009-08883 from the Ministryof Science and Innovation of Spain.

Author details

Francisco Mercado[1], Paloma Barjola[1], Marisa Fernández-Sánchez[1], Virginia Guerra[1] and Francisco Gómez-Esquer[2]

1 Department of Psychology, Faculty of Health Sciences, Rey Juan Carlos University, Madrid, Spain

2 Department of Anatomy and Human Embryology, Faculty of Health Sciences, Rey Juan Carlos University, Madrid, Spain

References

[1] Abeles, A., Pillinger, M., Solitar, B. and Abeles, M. (2007). Narrative Review: The Pathophysiology of Fibromyalgia. Annals of Internal Medicine 146, 726-734.

[2] Ablin, J., Neumann, L., Buskila, D. (2008). Pathogenesis of fibromyalgia – A review. Joint Bone Spine 75 (3), 273-279.

[3] Altamura, M., Elveväg, B., Blasi, G., Bertolino, A., Callicott, J.H., Weinberger D.R. et al. (2007). Dissociating the effects of Sternberg working memory demands in prefrontal cortex. Psychiatric Research 154, 103-114.

[4] Ambrose, K.R., Gracely R.H., Glass, J.M. (2012). Fibromyalgia dyscognition: concepts and issues. Rheumatismo 64 (4), 206-215.

[5] Apkarian, A.V., Bushnell, M.C., Treede, R.D., Zubieta, J.K. (2005). Human brain mechanisms of pain perception and regulation in health and disease. European Journal of Pain 9 (4), 463-484.

[6] Arnold, L.M., Crofford, L.J., Mease, P.J., Burgess, S.M., Palmer, S.C., Abetz, L., Martin, S.A. (2008). Patient perspectives on the impact of fibromyalgia. Patient Education and Counseling 73 (1), 114-120.

[7] Arnold, L.M., Hudson, J.I., Hess, E.V., Ware, A.E., Fritz, D.A., Auchenbach, M.B., Starck, L.O., Keck, P.E. Jr. (2004). Family study of fibromyalgia. Arthritis & Rheumatism 50 (3), 944-52.

[8] Baddeley, A. (2000). The episodic buffer: A new component of working memory? Trends in Cognitive Sciences 4, 417-423.

[9] Baliki, N., Schnitzer, T., Bauer, W. and Apkarian, V. (2011). Brain Morphological Signatures for Chronic Pain. Plos ONE 6 (10), 1-13.

[10] Baliki, M.N., Geha, P.Y., Apkarian, A.V., Chialvo, D.R. (2008). Beyond feeling: chronic pain hurts the brain, disrupting the default-mode network dinamics. The Journal of Neuroscience 28 (6), 1398-1403.

[11] Barbosa, F.R., Matsuda, J.B., Mazucato, M., de Castro França, S., Zingaretti, S.M., da Silva, L.M., Martinez-Rossi, N.M., Júnior, M.F., Marins, M., Fachin, A.L. (2012). Influence of catechol-O-methyltransferase (COMT) gene polymorphisms in pain sensibility of Brazilian fibromyalgia patients. Rheumatology International 32 (2), 427–430.

[12] Belfer, I., Segall, S. (2011). COMT genetic variants and pain. Drugs Today (Barc). 47 (6), 457-67.

[13] Bennett, R. (2005). Fibromyalgia: present to future. Current Rheumatology Reports 7, 371–376.

[14] Bondy, B., Spaeth, M., Offenbaecher, M., Glatzeder, K., Stratz, T., Schwarz, M., de Jonge, S., Krüger, M., Engel, R.R., Färber, L., Pongratz, D.E., Ackenheil, M. (1999). The T102C polymorphism of the 5-HT2A-receptor gene in fibromyalgia. Neurobiology of Disease 6 (5), 433-9.

[15] Bruder, G.E., Keilp, J.G., Xu, H., Shikhman, M., Schori, E., Gorman, J.M., Gilliam, T.C. (2005). Catechol-O-methyltransferase (COMT) genotypes and working memory: associations with differing cognitive operations. Biological Psychiatry 58 (11), 901-7.

[16] Bunge, S.A., Klingberg, T., Jacobsen, R.B., Gabrieli, J.D.E. (2000). A resource model of the neural basis of executive working memory. Proceedings of the National Academy of Sciences of the United States of America (PNAS) 97 (7), 3573-3578.

[17] Burgmer, M., Pogatzki-Zahn, E., Markus, G., Stüber, C., Wessoleck, E., Heuft, G., and Pfleiderer, B. (2010). Fibromyalgia unique temporal brain activation during experimental pain: a controlled fMRI Study. Journal Neural Transmission 117, 123-131.

[18] Burgmer, M., Pogatzki-Zahn, E., Gaubitz, M. Wessoleck, E., Heuft, G. Pfleiderer, B. (2009). Altered brain activity during pain processing in fibromyalgia. Neuroimage 44 (2), 502-508.

[19] Bushnell, M.C., Apkarian, A.V. (2005). Representation of pain in the brain. In: McMahon S, Koltzenburg M (eds). Textbook of pain, 5th edn. Churchill Livingstone, Philadelphia, pp. 267–289

[20] Buskila, D. (2009). Developments in the scientific and clinical understanding of fibromyalgia. Arthritis Research and Therapy 11 (5), 242-249.

[21] Buskila, D., Cohen, H., Neumann, L., Ebstein, R.P. (2004). An association between fibromyalgia and the dopamine D4 receptor exon III repeat polymorphism and relationship personality traits. Molecular Psychiatry 9 (8), 730-731.

[22] Buskila, D., Neumann, L., Hazanov, I., Carmi, R. (1996). Familial aggregation in the fibromyalgia syndrome. Seminars in Arthritis and Rheumatism 26 (3), 605-11.

[23] Buskila, D., Sarzi-Puttini, P., Ablin, J.N. (2007). The genetics of fibromyalgia syndrome. Pharmacogenomics 8 (1), 67-74.

[24] Carrillo-de-la-Peña, M.T., Vallet, M., Pérez, M.I., Gómez-Perretta, C. (2006). Intensity Dependence of Auditory-Evoked Cortical Potentials in Fibromyalgia Patients: A Test of the Generalized Hypervigilance Hypothesis. Journal of Pain 7, 480-487.

[25] Catapano, L.A., Manji, H.K. (2007). G protein-coupled receptors in major psychiatric disorders. Biochimica et Biophysica Acta 1768 (4), 976-93.

[26] Ceko, M., Bushnell, C. and Gracely, R. (2012). Neurobiology Underlying Fibromyalgia Symptoms. Pain Research and Treatment 2012, Article ID 585419, 8 pages

[27] Cifre, I., Sitges, C., Fraiman, D., Muñoz, M.A., Balenzuela, P., González-Roldán, A., Martínez-Jauand, M., Birbaumer, N., Chialvo, D.R., Montoya, P. (2012). Disrupted functional connectivity of the pain network in fibromyalgia. Psychosomatic Medicine 74 (1), 55-62.

[28] Cohen, H., Buskila, D., Neumann, L., Ebstein, R.P. (2002). Confirmation of an association between fibromyalgia and serotonin transporter promoter region (5- HTTLPR) polymorphism, and relationship to anxiety-related personality traits. Arthritis & Rheumatism 46 (3), 845-7.

[29] Cohen, H., Neumann, L., Glazer, Y., Ebstein, R.P., Buskila, D. (2009). The relationship between a common catechol-O-methyltransferase (COMT) polymorphism val(158) met and fibromyalgia. Clinical and Experimental Rheumatology 27 (5), 51-6.

[30] Cook, D.B., Lange, G., Ciccone, D.S., Liu, W.C., Steffener, J. Natelson B.H. (2004). Functional imaging of pain in patients with primary fibromyalgia. Journal of Rheumatology 31 (2), 364-378.

[31] Correa, A., Miró, E., Martínez, P., Sánchez, A. and Lupiáñez, J. (2011). Temporal preparation and inhibitory deficit in fibromyalgia síndrome. Brain and Cognition 75, 211-216.

[32] Craggs, J.G., Staud, R., Robinson, M.E., Perlstein, W.M., Price, D.D. (2012). Effective connectivity among brain regions associated with slow temporal summation of C-fiber-evoked pain in fibromyalgia patients and healthy controls. The Journal of Pain 13 (4), 390-400.

[33] Crombez, G., Van Damme, S., Eccleston, C. (2005). Hypervigilance to pain: An experimental and clinical analysis. Pain 116, 4-7.

[34] Dadabhoy, D., Crofford, L., Spaeth, M., Russell, J. and Clauw, D. (2008). Evidence-based biomarkers for fibromyalgia syndrome. Arthritis Research & Therapy 10 (211), 1-18.

[35] Dagher, A., Owen, A. M., Boecker, H., Brooks, D.J. (1999). Mapping the network for planning: A correlational PET activation study with the Tower of London task. Brain 122 (10), 1973-1987.

[36] Desmeules, J., Piguet, V., Besson, M., Chabert, J., Rapiti, E., Rebsamen, M., Rossier, M.F., Curtin, F., Dayer, P., Cedraschi, C. (2012). Psychological distress in fibromyalgia patients: A role for catechol-O-methyl-transferase Val158met polymorphism. Health Psychology 31 (2), 242-249.

[37] Diatchenko, L., Slade, G.D., Nackley, A.G., Bhalang, K., Sigurdsson, A., Belfer, I., Goldman, D., Xu, K., Shabalina, S.A., Shagin, D., Max, M.B., Makarov, S.S., Maixner, W. (2005). Genetic basis for individual variations in pain perception and the development of a chronic pain condition. Human Molecular Genetics 14 (1), 135-43.

[38] Diaz-Asper, C.M., Weinberger, D.R., Goldberg, T.E. (2006). Catechol-O-methyltransferase polymorphisms and some implications for cognitive therapeutics. NeuroRx 3 (1), 97-105.

[39] Dick, B.D., Verrier, M.J., Harker, K.T., and Rashiq, S. (2008). Disruption of cognitive function in fibromyalgia syndrome. Pain 139 (3), 610-616.

[40] Drenth, J.P., Waxman, S.G. (2007). Mutations in sodium-channel gene SCN9A cause a spectrum of human genetic pain disorders. The Journal of Clinical Investigation 117 (12), 3603–3609.

[41] Duschek, S., Werner, N.S., Winkelmann, A. Wankner, S. (2013). Implicit Memory Function in Fibromyalgia Syndrome. Behavioral Medicine 39 (1), 11-16.

[42] Emad, Y., Ragab, Y., Zeinhom, F., El-Khouly, G., Abou-Zeid, A., Rasker, J.J. (2008). Hippocampus dysfunction may explain symptoms of fibromyalgia syndrome. A study with single-voxel magnetic resonance spectroscopy. Journal of Rheumatology 35, 1371-1377.

[43] Fan, P.T. (2004). Fibromyalgia and chronic fatigue syndrome. APLAR Journal of Rheumatology 7 (3), 219-231.

[44] Fayed, N., García-Campayo, J., Magallón, R., Andrés-Bergareche, H., Luciano, JV., Andres, E., Beltrán, J. (2010). Localized 1H-NMR spectroscopy in patients with fibromyalgia: a controlled study of changes in cerebral glutamate/glutamine, inositol, choline, and N-acetylaspartate. Arthritis Research & Therapy 12 (4), R134.

[45] Fernández-de-Las-Peñas, C., Ambite-Quesada, S., Gil-Crujera, A., Cigarán-Méndez, M., Peñacoba-Puente, C. (2012). Catechol-O-methyltransferase Val158Met polymorphism influences anxiety, depression, and disability, but not pressure pain sensitivity, in women with fibromyalgia syndrome. The Journal of Pain 13 (11), 1068-74.

[46] Finan, P.H., Zautra, A.J., Davis, M.C., Lemery-Chalfant, K., Covault, J., Tennen, H. (2011). COMT moderates the relation of daily maladaptive coping and pain in fibromyalgia. Pain 152 (2), 300-307.

[47] Finan, P.H., Zautra, A.J., Davis, M.C., Lemery-Chalfant, K., Covault, J., Tennen, H. (2010). Genetic influences on the dynamics of pain and affect in fibromyalgia. Health Psychology 29 (2), 134-142.

[48] Frank, B., Niesler, B., Bondy, B., Späth, M., Pongratz, D.E., Ackenheil, M., Fischer, C., Rappold, G. (2004). Mutational analysis of serotonin receptor genes: HTR3A and HTR3B in fibromyalgia patients. Clinical Rheumatology 23 (4), 338-344.

[49] García-Campayo, J., Fayed, N., (2010). Clinical Magnetic Resonance Neuroimaging in Fibromyalgia. Neuroimaging, Cristina Marta Del-Ben (Ed.), 111-124.

[50] García-Fructuoso, F.J., Lao-Villadóniga, J.I., Beyer, K., Santos, C. (2006). Relationship between COMT gene genotypes and the severity of fibromyalgia. Reumatología Clínica 2 (4), 168–172.

[51] Geisser, M.E., Glass, J.M., Rajcevska, L.D., Clauw, D.J., Williams, D.A., Kileny, P.R., and Gracely, R.H. (2008). A Psychophysical Study of Auditory and Pressure Sensitivity in Patients With Fibromyalgia and Healthy Controls. Journal of Pain 9, 417-422.

[52] Giesecke, T., Gracely, R.H., Williams, D.A., Geisser, M.E., Petzke, F.W. (2005). The relationship between depression, clinical pain, and experimental pain in a chronic pain cohort. Arthritis and Rheumatism 52 (5), 1577-1584.

[53] Glass, J.M., Williams, D.A., Fernández-Sánchez, M.L., Kairys, A., Barjola, P., Heitzeg, M.M., Clauw, D.J., and Schmidt-Wilcke, T. (2011). Executive Function in Chronic Pain Patients and Healthy Controls: Different Cortical Activation During Response Inhibition in Fibromyalgia. The Journal of Pain 12 (12), 1219-1229.

[54] Glass, J.M. (2010). Cognitive dysfunction in fibromyalgia syndrome. Journal of Musculoskeletal Pain 18 (4), 367-372.

[55] Glass, J.M. (2009). Review of cognitive dysfunction in fibromyalgia: a convergence on working memory and attentional control impairments. Rheumatic Diseases Clinics of North America 35 (2), 299-311.

[56] Glass, J.M. (2006). Cognitive dysfunction in fibromyalgia and chronic fatigue syndrome: new trends and future directions. Current Rheumatology Reports 8 (6), 425-429.

[57] Glass, J.M., Park, D.C., Minear, M., and Crofford, L.J. (2005). Memory beliefs and function in fibromyalgia patients. Journal Psychosomatic Research 58, 263- 269.

[58] Glass, J.M., Park, D.C. (2001). Cognitive dysfunction in fibromyalgia. Current Rheumatology Reports 3 (2), 123-127.

[59] Gómez-Esquer, F., Barjola, P., Fernández-Sánchez, M., Mercado, F. (2012). Dopamine D2 receptor polymorphism influence on working memory functioning in Fibromyalgia. 14th World Congress on Pain – International Association for the Study of Pain (IASP)

[60] González, J.L., Mercado, F., Barjola, P., Carretero, I., Lopez-Lopez, A., Bullones, M.A., Fernandez-Sanchez, M., Alonso, M. (2010). Generalized hypervigilance in fibromyalgia patients: an experimental analysis with the emotional Stroop paradigm. Journal Psychosomatic Research 69, 279-287.

[61] Grace, G., Nielson, W., Hopkins, M. and Berg, M. (1999) . Concentration and Memory Deficits in Patients with Fibromyalgia Syndrome. Journal of Clinical and Experimental Neuropsychology 21 (4), 477-487.

[62] Gracely, R.H., Ambrose, K.R. (2011). Neuroimaging of fibromyalgia. Best Practice and Research: Clinical Rheumatology 25 (2), 271-284.

[63] Gracely, R.H., Geisser, M.E., Giesecke, T., Grant, M.A., Petzke, F. Williams, D.A. et al. (2004). Pain catastrophizing and neural responses to pain among persons with fibromyalgia. Brain 127 (4), 835-843.

[64] Gracely, R.H., Petzke, F., Wolf, J.M., and Clauw, D.J. (2002). Functional magnetic resonance imaging evidence of augmented pain processing in fibromyalgia. Arthritis and Rheumatism 46 (5), 1333-1343.

[65] Graven-Nielsen, T., Aspegren Kendall, S., Henriksson, K.G., Bengtsson, M., Sorensen, J., Johnson, A., Gerdle, B., Arendt-Nielsen, L. (2000). Ketamine reduces muscle pain, temporal summation, and referred pain in fibromyalgia patients. Pain 85, 483-491.

[66] Grisart, J., Van del Linden, M. and Masquelier, E. (2002). Controlled processes and automaticity in memory functioning in Fobromyalgia patienes: relation with emotional distress and hypervigilance. Journal of Clinical and Experimental Neuropsychology 24 (8), 994-1009.

[67] Gupta, A., Silman, A.J. (2004). Psychological stress and fibromyalgia: a review of the evidence suggesting a neuroendocrine link. Arthritis Research & Therapy 6 (3), 98-106.

[68] Gursoy, S. (2002). Absence of association of the serotonin transporter gene polymorphism with the mentally healthy subset of fibromyalgia patients. Clinical Rheumatology 21 (3), 194-197.

[69] Harris, R.E. (2010). Elevated excitatory neurotransmitter levels in the fibromyalgia brain. Arthritis Research & Therapy 12 (5), 141.

[70] Harris, R.E., Sundgren, P.C., Craig, A.D., Kirshenbaum, E., Sen, A., Napadow, V., Clauw, D.J. (2009). Elevated insular glutamate in fibromyalgia is associated with experimental pain. Arthritis & Rheumatism 60 (10), 3146-3152.

[71] Harris, R.E., Sundgren, P.C., Pang, Y., Hsu, M., Petrou, M., Kim, S.H., McLean, S.A., Gracely, R.H., Clauw, D.J. (2008). Dynamic levels of glutamate within the insula are associated with improvements in multiple pain domains in fibromyalgia. Arthritis & Rheumatism 58 (3), 903-907.

[72] Herrero, J.F., Laird, J.M., Lopez-García JA. (2000). Wind-up of spinal cord neurones and pain sensation: much ado about something? Progress Neurobiology 61, 169–203.

[73] Hosák, L. (2007). Role of the COMT gene Val158Met polymorphism in mental disorders: a review. European Psychiatry 22 (5), 276-281.

[74] Hsu, M.C., Harris, R.E., Sundgren, P.C., Welsh, R.C., Fernandes, C.R., Clauw, D.J., Williams, D.A. (2009). No consistent difference in gray matter volume between individuals with fibromyalgia and age-matched healthy subjects when controlling for affective disorder. Pain 143 (3), 262-267.

[75] Iannetti, G.D., Mouraux, A. (2010). From the neuromatrix to the pain matrix (and back). Experimental Brain Research 205 (1), 1-12.

[76] Julien, N., Goffaux, P., Arsenault, P., Marchand, S. (2005). Widespread pain in fibromyalgia is related to a deficit of endogenous pain inhibition. Pain 114, 295-302.

[77] Karoum, F., Chrapusta, S.J., Egan, M.F. (1994). 3-Methoxytyramine is the major metabolite of released dopamine in the rat frontal cortex. Journal of Neurochemistry 63 (3), 972-979.

[78] Katz, R.S., Heard, A.R., Mills, M., Leavitt, F. (2004). The prevalence and clinical impact of reported cognitive difficulties (fibrofog) in patients with rheumatic disease with and without fibromyalgia. Journal Clinical Rheumatology 10 (2), 53–58.

[79] Seong-Ho, K, Sang-Hyon, K, Seong-Kyu, K, Eun Jung, N, SeungWoo, H &SeungJae, L. (2012). Spatial versus verbal memoryimpairments in patientswithfibromyalgia Rheumatology Int 32, 1135-1142

[80] Kosek, E., Hansson, P. (1997). Modulatory influence on somatosensory perception from vibration and heterotopic noxious conditioning stimulation (HNCS) in fibromyalgia patients and healthy subjects. Pain 70, 41-51.

[81] Kuchinad, A., Schweinhardt, P., Seminowicz, D.A., Wood, P.B., Chizh, B.A., and Bushnell, M.C. (2007). Accelerated brain gray matter loss in fibromyalgia patients: premature aging of the brain? The Journal of Neuroscience 27 (15), 4004-4007.

[82] Kwiatek, R., Barnden, L., Tedman, R., Jarrett, R., Chew, J., Rowe, C. and Pile, K. (2000). Regional cerebral blood flow in fibromyalgia: Single-photon–emission computed tomography evidence of reduction in the pontine tegmentum and thalami. Arthritis and Rheumatism 43 (12), 2823–2833.

[83] Landro, N.I., Stiles, T.C., Sletvold, H. (1997). Memory functioning in patients with primary fibromyalgia and major depression and healthy controls. Journal Psychosomatic Research 42 (3), 297–306.

[84] Laruelle, M. (1998). Imaging dopamine transmission in schizophrenia. A review and meta-analysis. The Quarterly Journal of Nuclear Medicine 42 (3), 211-221.

[85] Lautenbacher, S., Rollman GB. (1997). Possible deficiencies of pain modulation in fibromyalgia. Clinical Journal of Pain 13, 189-196.

[86] Leavitt, F, &Katz, R.S. (2008). Speed of Mental Operations in Fibromyalgia: A SelectiveNamingSpeedDeficit Journal of Clinical Rheumatology 14 (4), 214-218

[87] Leavitt, F., Katz, R.S. (2006). Distraction as a key determinant of impaired memory in patients with fibromyalgia. The Journal of Rheumatology 33 (1), 127-132.

[88] Lee, Y.H., Choi, S.J., Ji, J.D., Song, G.G. (2012). Candidate gene studies of fibromyalgia: a systematic review and meta-analysis. Rheumatology International 32 (2), 417-426.

[89] Lee, Y.C., Nassikas, N.J., Clauw, D.J. (2011). The role of the central nervous system in the generation and maintenance of chronic pain in rheumatoid arthritis, osteoarthritis and fibromyalgia. Arthritis Research & Therapy 13 (2), 211-221.

[90] Legrain, V., Iannetti, G.D., Plaghki, L., Mouraux, A. (2011). The pain matrix reloaded: A salience detection system for the body. Progress in Neurobiology 93 (1), 111-124.

[91] Lorenz, J., Minoshima, S., Casey, K.L. (2003). Keeping pain out of mind: the role of the dorsolateral prefrontal cortex in pain modulation. Brain 126 (5), 1079-1091.

[92] Lotta, T., Vidgren, J., Tilgmann, C., Ulmanen, I., Melén, K., Julkunen, I., Taskinen, J. (1995). Kinetics of human soluble and membrane-bound catechol O-methyltransferase: a revised mechanism and description of the thermolabile variant of the enzyme. Biochemistry 34 (13), 4202-4210.

[93] Luerding, R., Weigand, T., Bogdahn, U., and Schmidt-Wilcke, T. (2008). Working memory performance is correlated with local brain morphology in the medial frontal and anterior cingulate cortex in fibromyalgia patients: structural correlates of pain–cognition interaction. Brain 131 (12), 3222-3231.

[94] Lutz, J., Jäger, L., de Quervain, D., Krauseneck, T., Padberg, F., Wichnalek, M., Beyer, A., Stahl, R., Zirngibl, B., and Morhard, D. (2008). White and gray matter abnormalities in the brain of patients with fibromyalgia: A diffusion-tensor and volumetric imaging study. Arthritis and Rheumatism 58 (12), 3960-3969.

[95] Maestú, C., Cortes, A., Vazquez, J.M., del Rio, D., Gomez-Arguelles, J.M., del Pozo, F., Nevado, A. (2013). Increased brain responses during subjectively-matched mechanical pain stimulation in fibromyalgia patients as evidenced by MEG. Clinical Neurophysiology 124 (4), 752-760.

[96] Malt, E.A., Olafsson, S., Aakvaag, A., Lund, A., Ursin, H. (2003). Altered dopamine D2 receptor function in fibromyalgia patients: a neuroendocrine study with buspirone in women with fibromyalgia compared to female population based controls. Journal of Affective Disorders 75 (1), 77-82.

[97] Martínez-Jauand, M., Sitges, C., Rodríguez, V., Picornell, A., Ramon, M., Buskila, D., Montoya, P. (2013). Pain sensitivity in fibromyalgia is associated with catechol-O-methyltransferase (COMT) gene. European Journal of Pain 17 (1), 16-27.

[98] Martínez-Lavín M. (2004). Fibromyalgia as a sympathetically maintained pain syndrome. Current Pain Headache Reports 8, 385-389.

[99] Matsuda, J.B., Barbosa, F.R., Morel, L.J., et al. (2010). Serotonin receptor (5-HT 2A) and catechol-O-methyltransferase (COMT) gene polymorphisms: triggers of fibromyalgia? Revista Brasileira de Reumatologia 50 (2), 141-149.

[100] Mease, P.J., Arnold, L.M., Crofford, L.J., Williams, D.A., Russell, I.J., Humphrey, L., Abetz, L., and Martin, S.A. (2008). Identifying the clinical domains of fibromyalgia: contributions from clinician and patient Delphi exercises. Arthritis & Rheumatism 59, 952-960.

[101] Mercado, F., Gonzalez, J.L., Barjola, P., Fernández-Sánchez, M., López-López, A., Alonso, M., and Gómez-Esquer, F. (in press). Brain correlates of cognitive inhibition in Fibromyalgia: Emotional intrusion of symptom-related words. International Journal of Psychophysiology.

[102] Mercado, F., Barjola, P., Fernández-Sánchez, M., Dragoi, D., Fresno, V., Cardoso, S., Gómez-Esquer, F. (submitted). Evidence of altered working memory processes in fibromyalgia patients: an event-related potential study. Pain

[103] Montoya, P., Sitges, C., García-Herrera, M., Izquierdo, R., Truyols, M., Blay, N., and Collado, D. (2005) Abnormal Affective Modulation of Somatosensory Brain Processing Among Patients With Fibromyalgia. Psychsomatic Medicine 67, 957-963.

[104] Montoya, P., Larbig, W., Braun, C., Preissl, H., Birbaumer, N. (2004). Influence of Social Support and Emotional Context on Pain Processing and Magnetic Brain Responses in Fibromyalgia. Arthritis & Rheumatism 50 (12), 4035-4044.

[105] Munguia-Izquierdo, D., Legaz-Arrese, A., Moliner-Urdiales, D., Reverter-Masia, J. (2008). Neuropsychological performance in patients with fibromyalgia syndrome: relation to pain and anxiety. Psicothema 20, 427-431.

[106] Muñoz-Céspedes, J.M., Tirapu-Ustárroz, J. (2001). Rehabilitación Neuropsicológica. Ed. Síntesis.

[107] Napadow, V., Kim, J., Clauw, D. and Harris, R. (2012) Decreased Intrinsic Brain Connectivity Is Associated With Reduced Clinical Pain in Fibromyalgia. Arthritis & Rheumatism, 64 (7), 2398-2403.

[108] Napadow, V., LaCount, L., Park, K., As-Sanie, S., Clauw, D.J., Harris, R.E. (2010). Intrinsic brain connectivity in fibromyalgia is associated with chronic pain intensity. Arthritis and Rheumatism 62 (8), 2545-2555.

[109] Okifuji, A., Turk, DC. (2002). Stress and psychophysiological dysregulation in pa-
       tients with fibromyalgia syndrome. Applied Psychophysiology and Biofeedback 27,
       129-141.

[110] Offenbaecher, M., Bondy, B., de Jong, S., Glatzeder, K., Kruger, M., Schoeps, P., Ac-
       kenheil, M. (1999). Possible association of fibromyalgia with a polymorphism in the
       serotonin transporter gene regulatory region. Arthritis and Rheumatism 42 (11),
       2482-2488.

[111] Park, D.C., Glass, J.M., Minear, M., Crofford, L.J. (2001). Cognitive function in fibro-
       myalgia patients. Arthritis & Rheumatism 44 (9), 2125-2133.

[112] Peyron, R., Laurent, B., García-Larrea, L. (2000). Functional imaging of brain respons-
       es to pain. A review and meta-analysis. Neurophysiologie Clinique 30 (5), 263-288.

[113] Potvin, S., Larouche, A., Normand, E., de Souza, J.B., Gaumond, I., Grignon, S.,
       Marchand, S. (2009). DRD3 Ser9Gly polymorphism is related to thermal pain percep-
       tion and modulation in chronic widespread pain patients and healthy controls. The
       Journal of Pain 10 (9), 969-975.

[114] Potvin, S., Larouche, A., Normand, E., de Souza, J.B., Gaumond, I., Marchand, S.,
       Grignon, S. (2010). No relationship between the ins del polymorphism of the seroto-
       nin transporter promoter and pain perception in fibromyalgia patients and healthy
       controls. European Journal of Pain 14 (7), 742-746.

[115] Price, D.D., Staud, R., Robinson, M.E., Mauderli, A.P., Cannon, R., Vierck, C.J. (2002).
       Enhanced
       temporal summation of second pain and its central modulation in
       fibromyalgia patients. Pain 99, 49-59.

[116] Pujol, J., López-Solá, M., Ortiz, H., Vilanova, J.C., Harrison, B.J. Yücel, M., Soriano-
       Mas, C., Cardoner, N. Deus, J. (2009). Mapping brain response to pain in fibromyal-
       gia patients using temporal analysis of fMRI. PLoS One 4 (4), e5224.

[117] Reyes del Paso G.A., Pulgar A., Duschek S., Garrido S. (2012). Cognitive impairment
       in fibromyalgia syndrome: the impact of cardiovascular regulation, pain, emotional
       disorders and medication. European Journal of Pain 16, 421-429.

[118] Robinson, M.E., Craggs, J.G., Price, D.D., Perlstein, W.M., Staud, R. (2011). Gray mat-
       ter volumes of pain-related brain areas are decreased in fibromyalgia syndrome. The
       Journal of Pain 12 (4), 436-443.

[119] Rolls, E.T., O'Doherty, J., Kringelbach, M.L., Francis, S., Bowtell, R., McGlone, F.
       (2003). Representations of pleasant and painful touch in the human orbitofrontal and
       cingulate cortices. Cerebral Cortex 13 (3), 308-317.

[120] Russell, I.J., Orr, M.D., Littman, B., Vipraio, G.A., Alboukrek, D., Michalek, J.E., et al.
       (1994). Elevated cerebrospinal fluid levels of substance P in patients with the fibro-
       myalgia syndrome. Arthritis and Rheumatism 37, 1593-1601.

[121] Russell, I.J., Vaeroy, H., Javors, M., Nyberg, F. (1992). Cerebrospinal fluid biogenic amine metabolites in fibromyalgia/fibrositis syndrome and rheumatoid arthritis. Arthritis and Rheumatism 35, 550-556.

[122] Sawamoto, N., Honda, M., Okada, T., Hanakawa, T., Kanda, M., Fukuyama, H., Konishi, J., Shibasaki, H. (2000). Expectation of pain enhances responses to nonpainful somatosensory stimulation in the anterior cingulate cortex and parietal operculum/ posterior insula: an event-related functional magnetic resonance imaging study. The Journal of Neuroscience 20 (19), 7438-7445.

[123] Schmidt-Wilcke, T., Clauw, D.J. (2010). Pharmacotherapy in fibromyalgia (FM) – Implications for the underlying pathophysiology. Pharmacology & Therapeutics 127 (3), 283-294.

[124] Schmidt-Wilcke, T., Luerding, R., Weigand, T., Jürgens, T., Schuierer, G., Leinisch, E., Bogdahn, U. (2007). Striatal grey matter increase in patients suffering from fibromyalgia – a voxel-based morphometry study. Pain 132 (1), 109-116.

[125] Schweinhardt, P., Sauro, K.M. Bushnell, C. (2008). Fibromyalgia: a disorder of the brain? The Neuroscientist 14 (5), 415-421.

[126] Seminowicz, D.A., Davis, K.D. (2007). Pain enhances functional connectivity of a brain network evoked by performance of a cognitive task. Journal of Neurophysiology 97 (5), 3651-3659.

[127] Seo., J. Kim, S.H., Kim, Y.T., Song, H.J., Lee, J.J., Kim, S.H., Han, S.W., Nam, E.J., Kim, S.K., Lee, H.J., Lee, S.J., Chang, Y. (2012). Working memory impairment in fibromyalgia patients associated with altered frontoparietal memory network. PLoS One 7 (6), e37808.

[128] Singer, T., Seymour, B., O'Doherty, J., Kaube, H., Dolan, R.J., Frith, C.D. (2004). Empathy for pain involves the affective but not sensory components of pain. Science 303 (5661), 1157-1162.

[129] Small, K.M., McGraw, D.W., Liggett, S.B. (2003). Pharmacology and physiology of human adrenergic receptor polymorphisms. Annual Review of Pharmacology and Toxicology 43, 381-411.

[130] Smith, S.B., Maixner, D.W., Fillingim, R.B., Slade, G., Gracely, R.H., Ambrose, K., Zaykin, D.V., Hyde, C., John, S., Tan, K., Maixner, W., Diatchenko, L. (2012). Large candidate gene association study reveals genetic risk factors and therapeutic targets for fibromyalgia. Arthritis and Rheumatism 64 (2), 584-93.

[131] Solberg, L., Carlson, C., Crofford, L., Leeuw, R. and Segerstrom, S. (2010). Self-regulatory deficits in fibromyalgia and temporomandibular disorders. Pain 151, 37-44.

[132] Stahl, S.M. (2009). Fibromyalgia – pathways and neurotransmitters. Human Psychopharmacology and Clinical Experiment 24 (1), 11-17.

[133] Staud, R., Price, D.D., Robinson, M.E., Mauderli, A.P., Vierck, C.J. (2004). Mainte-
        nance of windup of second pain requires less frequent stimulation in fibromyalgia
        patients compared to normal controls. Pain 110 (3), 689-696.

[134] Staud, R. Cannon R.C., Mauderli, A.P., Robinson, M.E., Price, D.D., Vierck, C.J., Jr.
        (2003). Temporal summation of pain from mechanical stimulation of muscle tissue in
        normal controls and subjects with fibromyalgia syndrome. Pain 102, 87-95.

[135] Suhr, J. (2003). Neuropsychological impairment in fibromyalgia Relation to depres-
        sion, fatigue, and pain. Journal of Psychsomatic Research 55, 321-329.

[136] Tagliazucchi, E., Balenzuela, P., Fraiman, D., Chialvo, D.R. (2010). Brain resting state
        is disrupted in chronic back pain patients. Neuroscience letters 485 (1), 26-31.

[137] Thieme, K., Spies, C., Sinha, P., Turk, D.C., Flor, H., 2005. Predictors of pain behav-
        iors in fibromyalgia syndrome. Arthritis and Rheumatism 53, 343–350.

[138] Tracey, I., Johns, E. (2010). The pain matrix: reloaded or reborn as we image tonic
        pain using arterial spin labelling. Pain 148 (3), 359-360.

[139] Tracey, I., Mantyh P.W. (2007). The cerebral signature for pain perception and its
        modulation. Neuron 55 (3), 377-391.

[140] Treister, R., Pud, D., Ebstein, R.P., Laiba, E., Gershon, E., Haddad, M., Eisenberg, E.
        (2009). Associations between polymorphisms in dopamine neurotransmitter path-
        way genes and pain response in healthy humans. Pain 147 (1-3), 187-193.

[141] Valdés, M., Collado, A., Bargalló, N., Vázquez, M., Rami, L., Gómez, E., Salamero, M.
        (2010). Increased glutamate/glutamine compounds in the brains of patients with fi-
        bromyalgia: a magnetic resonance spectroscopy study. Arthritis and Rheumatism 62
        (6), 1829-1836.

[142] Valet, M., Sprenger, T., Boecker, H., Willoch, F., Rummeny, E., Conrad, B., Erhard, P.,
        Tolle, TR. (2004). Distraction modulates connectivity of the cingulo-frontal cortex and
        the midbrain during pain – an fMRI analysis. Pain 109 (3), 399-408.

[143] Vargas-Alarcón, G., Álvarez-León, E., Fragoso, J.M., Vargas, A., Martínez, A., Vallejo,
        M., Martínez-Lavín, M. (2012). A SCN9A gene-encoded dorsal root ganglia sodium
        channel polymorphism associated with severe fibromyalgia. BMC Musculoskeletical
        Disorders 20, 13-28.

[144] Vargas-Alarcón, G., Fragoso, J.M., Cruz-Robles, D., Vargas, A., Martínez, A., Lao-Vil-
        ladóniga, J.I., García-Fructuoso, F., Vallejo, M., Martínez-Lavín, M. (2009). Associa-
        tion of adrenergic receptor gene polymorphisms with different fibromyalgia
        syndrome domains. Arthritis and Rheumatism 60 (7), 2169-2173.

[145] Vargas-Alarcón, G., Fragoso, J.M., Cruz-Robles, D., Vargas, A., Vargas, A., Lao-Villa-
        dóniga, J.I., García-Fructuoso, F., Ramos-Kuri, M., Hernández, F., Springall, R., Boja-
        lil, R., Vallejo, M., Martínez-Lavín, L. (2007). Catechol-O-methyltransferase gene

haplotypes in Mexican and Spanish patients with fibromyalgia. Arthritis Research & Therapy 9 (5), R110.

[146] Veldhuijzen, D., Sondaal, S. and Oosterman, J. (2012). Intact Cognitive Inhibition in Patients With Fibromyalgia but Evidence of Declined Processing Speed. The Journal of Pain 13 (5), 507-515.

[147] Verdejo-Garcia, A., Lopez-Torrecillas, F., Calandre, E.P., Delgado-Rodriguez, A., Bechara, A. (2009). Executive function and decision-making in women with fibromyalgia. Archives of Clinical Neuropsychology 24 (1), 113-122.

[148] Vierck, C.J. (2006). Mechanisms underlying development of spatially distributed chronic pain (fibromyalgia). Pain 124 (3), 242-263.

[149] Walteros, C., Sánchez-Navarro, J.P., Muñoz, M.A., Martínez-Selva, J.M., Chialvo, D., and Montoya, P. (2011). Altered associative learning and emotional decision making in fibromyalgia. Journal of Psychosomatic Research 70 (3), 294-301.

[150] Wiech, K., Seymour, B., Kalisch, R., Stephan, K.E., Koltzenburg, M., Driver, J., Dolan, R.J. (2005). Modulation of pain processing in hyperalgesia by cognitive demand. Neuroimage 27 (1), 59-69.

[151] Wiech, K, Ploner, M, & Tracey, I. (2008). Neurocognitive aspects of pain perception. Cell 12 (8), 306-313

[152] Williams, D.A., Clauw, D.J., Glass, J. (2011). Perceived Cognitive Dysfunction in Fibromyalgia Syndrome. Journal of Musculoskeletal Pain 19 (2), 66-75.

[153] Woolf, C.J. (2004). Pain: moving from symptom control toward mechanism-specific pharmacologic management. Annual International Medicin, 140, 441-451.

[154] Wolfe, F., Clauw, D.J., Fitzcharles, M.A., Goldenberg, D.L., Katz, R.S., Mease, P., Russell, A.S., Russell, I.J., Winfield, J.B., Yunus, M.B. (2010). The American College of Rheumatology preliminary diagnostic criteria for fibromyalgia and measurement of symptom severity. Arthritis Care & Research (Hoboken) 62 (5), 600-610.

[155] Wolfe, F., Smythe, H.A., Yunus, M.B., Bennett, R.M., Bombardier, C., Goldenberg, D.L., Tugwell, P., Campbell, S.M., Abeles, M., Clark, P. (1990). The American College of Rheumatology 1990 Criteria for the Classification of Fibromyalgia. Report of the Multicenter Criteria Committee. Arthritis and Rheumatism 33 (2), 160-172.

[156] Wood, P.B., Glabus, M.F., Simpson, R., Patterson, J.C., 2nd. (2009). Changes in gray matter density in fibromyalgia: correlation with dopamine metabolism. The Journal of Pain 10 (6), 609-618.

[157] Wood, P.B. (2008). Role of central dopamine in pain and analgesia. Expert Review of Neurotherapeutics 8 (5), 781-797.

[158] Wood, P.B., Patterson, I., James, C., Sunderland, J.J., Tainter, K.H., Glabus, M.F., Lilien, D.L. (2007b). Reduced presynaptic dopamine activity in fibromyalgia syndrome

demonstrated with positron emission tomography: a pilot study. The Journal of Pain 8 (1), 51-58.

[159] Wood, P.B., Schweinhardt, P., Jaeger, E., Dagher, A., Hakyemez, H., Rabiner, E.A., Bushnell, M.C., Chizh, B.A. (2007a). Fibromyalgia patients show an abnormal dopamine response to pain. The Journal of Neuroscience 25 (12), 3576-3582.

[160] Xiao, Y., He, W., Russell, I.J. (2011). Genetic polymorphisms of the beta2-adrenergic receptor relate to guanosine protein-coupled stimulator receptor dysfunction in fibromyalgia syndrome. The Journal of Rheumatology 38 (6), 1095-1103.

[161] Zhang, Y., Bertolino, A., Fazio, L., Blasi, G., Rampino, A., Romano, R., Lee, M.L., Xiao, T., Papp, A., Wang, D., Sadée, W. (2007). Polymorphisms in human dopamine D2 receptor gene affect gene expression, splicing, and neuronal activity during working memory. Proceedings of the National Academy of Sciences of the United States of America 104 (51), 20552-20557.

[162] Zubieta, J.K., Heitzeg, M.M., Smith, Y.R., et al. (2003). COMT val158met genotype affects mu-opioid neurotransmitter responses to a pain stressor. Science 299 (5610), 1240–1243.

Chapter 7

Quantitative Mapping of Angiogenesis by Magnetic Resonance Imaging

Teodora-Adriana Perles-Barbacaru and
Hana Lahrech

Additional information is available at the end of the chapter

1. Introduction

Since tumors are commonly associated with angiogenesis and compromised vascular wall integrity, the ability to focus noninvasive imaging techniques on vascular characteristics provides a physiologically-specific approach to tumor delineation which is of utility in guiding the biopsy and in surgical or radiation treatment planning. Hypervascularisation mapped by magnetic resonance imaging (MRI) correlates with histologically-assessed tumor grade [1]. It is also of value in distinguishing residual or recurrent tumor from treatment effects such as radiation induced necrosis [2]. Furthermore, by quantitatively assessing tumor vascularity and endothelial permeability, these approaches allow the evaluation of novel anti-angiogenic therapies, guiding drug development through preclinical stages, and facilitate the inter- and intra-subject comparisons. They also allow the assessment of the biological efficacy of therapies in the clinical setting, before more traditional criteria, such as tumor size change, become apparent. This is particularly important with novel antiangiogenic agents to distinguish potential responders from nonresponders.

This chapter focuses on MRI techniques for angiogenesis assessment. In particular it describes a newly developed quantitative MRI technique for in vivo blood volume fraction mapping for preclinical and above all for clinical applications in neurooncology. The blood volume fraction is a biomarker for angiogenesis and has proven successful in mapping brain dysfunction and in testing drug efficacy. The described technique is compared with other magnetic resonance imaging techniques currently employed in the preclinical and clinical setting. Therefore, this chapter provides an overview of existing quantitative MRI techniques, briefly explains their basic principle, states their acquisition and postprocessing requirements, and compares their advantages and limits. Quantitative results for blood volume fraction measures in laboratory animals and human subjects are presented and compared. Pitfalls and possibilities in neuro-oncological applications are pointed out and discussed.

2. When and why do we need to image angiogenesis?

The vasculature of brain tissue is a complex entity having multiple functions and regulatory mechanisms. One of its functions is to maintain and adjust the blood supply to meet the energy demands of the brain tissue. Most adjustments occur at the microscopic level. Tissues with a high metabolic turnover are generally equipped with a more extensive network of microvessels. Tumor growth and metastasis depend on tumor-induced angiogenesis, i.e. cancer cells with increased metabolism attract and maintain a blood supply [3, 4].

Brain capillaries are composed of a unique and continuous layer of endothelial cells connected by adhesion proteins. In addition, pericytes and foot like processes of astrocytes surround the basal lamina. This forms a regulatory interface between the blood and the cerebral parenchyma: the blood brain barrier (BBB). It is impermeable to many water soluble macromolecules, including many drugs and magnetic resonance contrast agents (CAs). However, the BBB is disrupted in many pathologic processes that involve inflammation or neovascularisation such as tumor growth.

Angiogenesis in malignant tumor tissue is structurally and functionally different from physiologic angiogenesis occurring during fetal development or tissue repair. The microvascular architecture is characterized by tortuous vessels with varying diameter, abnormal branching pattern and blind ending protrusions. Fast growing tumor vasculature is usually immature and lacks the regulatory mechanisms and competent BBB. This leads to a heterogeneous perfusion with parts of the tumor that are hyperperfused due to high microvascular density, and other parts that are hypoperfused with a low proportion of functional vessels. Blood turbulence and stasis as well as endothelial dysfunction lead to thrombosis. Remaining vessels may enlarge in an effort to compensate for the reduced blood flow. The resulting tissue hypoxia triggers secretion of angiogenic factors which maintain the angiogenic process [5]. Hyperpermeability of the incompetent BBB to macromolecules leads to edema and increased interstitial pressure which in turn may impede delivery of therapeutic agents to the tumor tissue.

Figure 1 shows representative vessel sections from healthy rat brain tissue and an experimental brain tumor.

Along with the mitotic index, presence of necrotic areas, invasive potential and cell differentiation, angiogenesis has been recognized as one of the diagnostic criterions of malignancy in the World Health Organization (WHO) classification. Similar to the presence of mitosis and necrosis, vascular proliferation is significantly correlated to survival [6-10]. Although neuroradiologic features can be highly suggestive, diagnosis is based on histologic examination. Neuroradiologic mapping of angiogenesis is important to guide the biopsy needle to sample appropriate tissue. After grading is established neuroimaging techniques help to delineate the

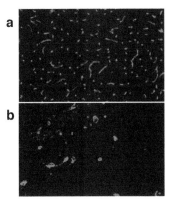

Figure 1. Immunofluorescent staining of collagen IV a component of the basal lamina of the vessel wall. a: Cortical vessels in a healthy rat are delicate, with a narrow distribution of vessel radii around 8 μm and randomly oriented and homogenously distributed. b: Tumor vasculature in a C6 glioma model is composed of sparse irregularly shaped and enlarged vessels. Parts of the tumor are not perfused.

tumor for radiotherapy and/or surgical planning. Magnetic resonance imaging (MRI) capable of multiparametric mapping and yielding high soft tissue contrast is widely used for diagnosis, surgical and radiation treatment planning as well as for treatment follow up. In many imaging facilities, perfusion MRI used to map vascular and hemodynamic parameters is part of the neuroimaging protocol, at least for diagnosis and treatment planning. In the advent of new treatment strategies targeted at the angiogenic process, noninvasive mapping of angiogenesis by MRI will become a requisite to monitor treatment efficacy in follow up studies.

3. What are imaging biomarkers of angiogenesis?

At the microscopic level, several parameters are used to describe and quantify the vascular network. Microvascular density, N_v (cm^{-2}), simply reports the number of vessels per unit area regardless of their shape, orientation or size. Together with the vascular volume density, which is the volume occupied by vascular walls and blood per unit volume of tissue, the microvascular density is the most frequently used parameter for angiogenesis quantification. The microvascular surface S_v is important for exchange processes between blood and interstitium and is approximately 100 cm^{2}g^{-1} tissue [11]. The length density L_v (cm^{-2}) is the total length of microvessels existing per unit volume of tissue. The vessel radii are important for rheological considerations because they define the cross sectional area that in turn is one of the parameters that determines the blood flow rate. The vascular area density is the ratio between the total area of vessel cross sections and the area of the region of interest (ROI) and correlates with the vascular volume density. The mean intercapillary distance in the human brain is about 40 μm [12] and is an index of the access of an interstitial cell to the exchange processes at the vascular boundary, since in the interstitium transport is mainly governed by diffusion. Other morphological parameters that change under physiologic and pathologic conditions exist, e. g. the tortuosity, interbranching distance, branching angle. Typical microvasculature from mouse cortex and tumor tissue is shown in Figure 12 b.

However MRI and other medical imaging techniques, such as computed tomography (CT) or positron emission tomography (PET) are rather macroscopic techniques. Obviously the above mentioned morphometric parameters of microvessels are not directly measurable. However, some hemodynamic parameters are accessible by these imaging techniques. One of them is the regional cerebral blood volume (CBV), which is the quantity of blood in ml per 100 g tissue that participates in the supply of oxygen and nutrients and in the discharge of toxic metabolites. It is often also expressed as a volume fraction (blood volume fraction, BVf), approximates the vascular volume density reported in microscopy studies and is related to the mean vascular diameter, the microvascular density and length density all of which are altered in the angiogenic process occurring in tumors. The conversion factor between both units is $100 \, \lambda/\varrho_{blood} \approx 93.75$ where λ is the brain-blood partition coefficient and ϱ_{blood} is the blood density [13]. CBV mapping has proven successful in assessing angiogenesis to study brain dysfunction and in testing drug efficacy.

Another parameter is the cerebral blood flow (CBF), which is the amount of blood arriving and leaving the tissue of interest in a time interval. The average CBF in humans is approximately 50 ml/min per 100g of brain tissue, while the critical threshold for neuronal function is approximately 20 ml/min per 100g. Another often reported quantity is the mean transit time (MTT), the average time required for blood to pass through the tissue volume of interest. It is related to CBV and CBF by MTT = CBV/CBF. Brain metabolism can be assessed by measuring the cerebral metabolic rate of oxygen ($CMRO_2$) which is about 130 µmol/min per 100g.

The permeability of the microvasculature to a substance is often reported as the product of the diffusional permeability coefficient P (cm min^{-1}) and the surface area S_v. PS_v has the unit of a volume flow per tissue mass (ml min^{-1} g^{-1}). Only values averaged over the volume of the voxel can be obtained without information about the morphology of the vasculature. Clinical studies have demonstrated the utility of this parameter for assessing malignancy and response to therapy in various tumors [14].

However, one MRI technique is sensitive to microvascular architecture, and the parameter obtained is called the vessel size index (VSI). This index is a weighted average of vessel sizes with a strong predominance of larger vessel sizes. It also depends on the vessel orientation which is assumed to be isotropic in healthy gray matter tissue, on the BVf and on the amount of contrast agent used.

Brain pathologies that are accompanied by vascular changes reflected by altered CBV, CBF, BBB permeability or combinations thereof, are brain infarction (ischemia) [15-17], multiple sclerosis [18, 19], infectious and inflammatory diseases [20], some forms of dementia such as Alzheimer's disease [21-23], acquired immune deficiency syndrome associated brain diseases [24, 25], and traumatic brain injury [26]. This chapter focuses on the quantification of tumor angiogenesis, which requires particular methodologic developments, due to the BBB permeability to most CAs.

4. Why are quantitative measures important?

Drugs targeting the angiogenic process such as inhibitors of angiogenic factors bring with them a need for an accurate means of assessing tumor angiogenesis and monitoring response to treatment. In the context of treatment monitoring comparison of values obtained at different time points are necessary. In the context of clinical trials comparisons between patients and centers need to be made.

Unfortunately, the signal intensity from most MR pulse sequences does not relate directly to any physiological parameter. Magnetic field strength, scanner parameters, sequence timing parameters, flip angle as well as image scaling, make the signal scanner dependent and comparisons between serial or multi-center studies difficult.

Procedures for data collection have to be found which are insensitive to scanner, sequence and operator influence, and which are reliable and reproducible over time and between patients. The measured parameters have to be examined for their biological meaning and related to clinically relevant quantities. In this way, changes at the microscopic level such as in cellular or microvascular structures can be detected as changes in MR parameters, such as relaxation times or magnetization transfer ratio, or as changes in diffusion and perfusion parameters at typical MR image resolutions of about 1 mm.

In theory, perfusion MRI techniques can yield quantitative hemodynamic parameters. To do so, they rely on a number of assumptions that are detailed below and require additional measurements that are either time consuming or invasive and therefore difficult in the clinical setting. In routine perfusion imaging, descriptive or semiquantitative parameters are therefore reported, some of which are discussed below. Typically, such values in the tissue of interest are reported relative to the corresponding value in a reference region, or are normalized to an average value taken from the literature. The reference region is chosen in healthy appearing brain tissue, usually in white matter or in the contralateral hemisphere symmetrical to the lesion. This is a pitfall when there is no reference region because the disease affects the whole brain such as a systemic cardiovascular pathology or a generalized infection, or when the "healthy appearing" reference region is affected by the disease, such as might occur with brain tumors that exert a mass effect, or have infiltrated the reference region.

5. What are the available quantitative magnetic resonance imaging techniques?

The perfusion MRI techniques that are presently used in the clinical practice are so called dynamic techniques. Dynamic techniques involve serial acquisition of MR images before, during and after the pass of an intravenously injected exogenous MRI CA through the tissue. As the CA enters into the tissue under investigation, the T_1 and T_2 values of tissue water decrease to an extent that is determined by the concentration of the CA.

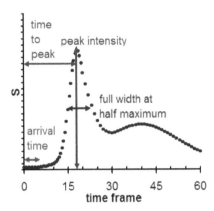

Figure 2. Characteristic signal intensity (S) time course during CA bolus passage. After the first high peak, the second peak corresponds to the second bolus passage after recirculation.

5.1. First pass or bolus tracking techniques

During the first pass of the CA bolus through the brain tissue the signal displays a characteristic intensity time course, which is related to the CA concentration in the tissue. Such a signal intensity time course is illustrated in Fig. 2 as an example of a positive (T_1 weighted) signal change. When changes in transverse relaxivity are exploited this technique is termed dynamic susceptibility contrast (DSC) MRI, which has superior signal to noise ratio (SNR) compared to T_1 weighted techniques. Mixed T_1 and T_2 weighting can complicate the interpretation. Fast imaging techniques with a recommended time resolution below 1.5 s are required, to adequately sample the signal dynamics. Even when using echo planar imaging (EPI) techniques, this requirement imposes limits to the spatial resolution and the number of slices that can be acquired.

Characteristic descriptive parameters measured form the observed signal changes during bolus pass include arrival time of the bolus, peak intensity, time to peak and full width at half maximum (Fig. 2). They generally depend on combinations of physiologic parameters, such as blood flow, fractional blood volume, and CA extravasation. Nevertheless, the peak signal amplitude was shown to correlate with the CBV [27].

For CBV quantification, the signal intensity during bolus pass is converted into a change in R_1 [28], R_2 or R_2^* [29] versus time reflecting the CA concentration. However, the proportionality constant between tissue relaxation rate change and CA concentration not only depends on CA properties and magnetic field strength. In particular the transverse relaxivity also depends on tissue properties such as microvascular architecture, vascular permeability, water exchange rate between intra- and extracellular compartment and blood oxygenation, all of which are spatially variable. The relaxivity is generally assumed to be the same as in plasma or venous blood. Any non-linearity between relaxation rate or signal change and CA concentration in tissue and blood will lead to errors [30].

In clinical routine, the CBV in the tissue of interest is given relative to a reference tissue. Maps of relative CBV are calculated by integrating the area under the CA concentration change during the first pass over time and since the CBV is calculated on the basis of signal recovery to the precontrast baseline, an adequate estimation of the baseline signal by signal averaging is essential. The accuracy of the CBV measure further depends on the ability to separate the first from the second pass of the CA (Fig "2). One approach to correct for CA recirculation is to fit a gamma variate function to the concentration versus time curve [31].

Tracer kinetic analysis [32] of the first bolus passage allows quantification of CBV, CBF and MTT, provided that the arterial CA concentration time course $(C_a(t))$, the so called arterial input function (AIF), is known.

The absolute CBV can be determined from the ratio of the areas under the tissue $C_{tissue}(t)$ and arterial CA concentration $C_a(t)$ versus time curves:

$$CBV = \frac{\int_{-\infty}^{\infty} C_{tissue}(t)dt}{\int_{-\infty}^{\infty} C_a(t)dt}$$

The tissue concentration versus time curve is the convolution of the tissue residue function $\Re(t)$ and the shape of the arterial concentration time curve $C_a(t)$ times the CBF:

$$C_{tissue}(t) = CBF \int_{-\infty}^{t} C_a(\tau)\Re(t-\tau)d\tau$$

$\Re(0)$ is equal to one at $t = 0$ when the CA enters the volume of interest. To calculate the CBF the impulse response CBF × $\Re(t)$ has to be determined by deconvolution, and then CBF is obtained as the initial ($t = 0$) height of the impulse response function.

The MTT is obtained by the central volume theorem: MTT = CBV/CBF

The AIF has to be specified from the major feeding artery. The imaging of the time course of the vascular CA concentration requires that the acquisition mode is insensitive to flow, that it has an adequate spatial resolution to identify a vessel and a high temporal resolution to sample the shape of the initial bolus passage. In addition, signal saturation for the very high vascular concentrations during the bolus peak has to be avoided. The AIF is difficult to obtain in a reliable way, and is the major source of error. It can be influenced by variations in injection conditions and by physiologic or morphologic parameters of the vasculature. Delay and dispersion occur from the site of the AIF measurement to the tissue ROI. Dispersion occurring in the larger vessels can be misinterpreted as a low tissue flow, although it is normal [33, 34]. The AIF measure is often affected by partial volume effects or suffers from saturation effects. Deconvolution methods [35, 36] have been proposed to provide more reliable absolute quantifications.

Most clinical studies using bolus tracking techniques report relative/semiquantitative results, because the determination of the AIF is considered too complex or inaccurate. When relative CBV values are reported, in addition to the above mentioned caveats regarding the choice of the reference region, the assumption of identical AIFs and of identical CA relaxivity in the compared tissue ROIs is made.

In the presence of CA leakage, CBV maps computed from T_2^* or T_2 weighted dynamic MRI tend to underestimate the CBV values, and may show false negative findings in the event of an active tumor recurrence [1]. Where T_1 weighted sequences are used, the presence of transendothelial CA leakage will act synergistically on signal intensity, causing artefactual CBV increases [37].

5.2. Dynamic contrast enhanced MRI

While with first pass techniques a vascular confinement of the CA is assumed, or models for leakage correction need to be applied, T_1 weighted dynamic contrast enhanced (DCE) MRI is designed to monitor the pharmacokinetics of the CA distribution within different compartments.

A simple qualitative or semiquantitative analysis of the signal enhancement curve with time after CA injection [38] use descriptors such as arrival time of the CA, maximum signal intensity or maximum intensity time ratio [39], initial uptake gradient or washout gradient. These parameters have a link to the underlying tissue physiology and CA pharmacokinetics, but the link is complex and not well defined. Unless the CA concentration versus time curves are used for semiquantitative analysis, they also depend on MR scaling factors.

For quantification, the time-varying signal has to be translated into tissue CA concentration. Pharmacokinetic modeling sets up a simplified description of tissue as a multi-compartment system. Although DCE MRI is used to quantify the microvascular permeability to the CA, appropriate kinetic models also allow quantification of the fractional volumes of the tissue compartments accessible to the CA: the CBV and the extravascular leakage volume assumed to be the extravascular extracellular compartment. CA transport between the compartments may then be modeled in terms of rate constants. Simple approaches model unidirectional CA flux (from intra- to extravascular compartments). More detailed approaches [40] recognize CA reflux in a bidirectional flux model. Kinetic modeling and interpretation is simplified by the assumption of a low extravasation rate compared to vascular flow rate (permeability limited model) preventing a decrease of the intravascular CA concentration [41]. When the CA extravasation rate is in the order of or higher than the blood flow rate in the vessel, the permeability limited model is no longer accurate. Flow limited extravasation is not unlikely in the case of tumor angiogenesis, since blood flow is perturbed and endothelial permeability is high. CAs of greater molecular weight help this limitation to be overcome, because their extravasation rate is lower.

The change in extravascular CA concentration dC_e/dt is proportional to the vascular permeability P (cm/min), the vascular surface area S_v (cm^2/g) and to the difference between the blood plasma concentration $C_p(t)$ (mM) and the extravascular concentration $C_e(t)$ and inversely proportional to the fractional volume of the extravascular compartment:

$$\frac{dC_e}{dt} = \frac{PS_v}{v_e}\left(C_p(t) - C_e(t)\right) \tag{1}$$

where ϱ is the tissue density and approximately 1 g/ml.

The CA concentration in the tissue $C_{tissue}(t)$ is composed of the concentrations in the plasma and in the extravascular compartment:

$$C_{tissue}(t) = v_p C_p(t) + v_e C_e(t) \tag{2}$$

where v_p is the fractional volume of the plasma compartment. The fractional plasma volume is related to the fractional blood volume (BVf) by: $v_p = (1\text{-Hct}) \, BVf$, where Hct is the capillary hematocrit.

Inserting Eq. 2 into Eq. 1 results in the following differential equation describing the CA flux across the endothelium where equal permeability for the outflux and the backflux is assumed:

$$\frac{dC_{tissue}}{dt} - v_p \frac{dC_p}{dt} = PS_v \varrho \left[C_p(t) - \frac{1}{v_e}(C_{tissue}(t) - v_p C_p(t)) \right] \tag{3}$$

The tissue concentration is given by the solution to Eq. 3:

$$C_{tissue}(t) = K^{trans} \int_0^t C_p(\tau) \exp[-k_{ep}(t-\tau)] d\tau + v_p C_p(t).$$

where $K^{trans} = PS_v \varrho$ is the coefficient of endothelial permeability and where the rate constant $k_{ep} = K^{trans}/v_e$ governs the backflux of CA into the vessel. The parameters in this expression can be fitted to the corresponding DCE-MRI data [42].

To derive the physiological parameters K^{trans}, v_e and v_p, the plasma concentration versus time $C_p(t)$ (the AIF) has to be measured or modeled. Tofts and Kermode [41] assumed a typical biexponential decay of C_p, due to rapid leakage into the extravascular extracellular compartment in extracerebral tissues and to the slower filtration by the kidneys. Larsson et al [43] measured it from serial blood samples, while Brix et al [44] included the plasma clearance rate as a free parameter in the fit.

Assumptions common to all models described here are the homogeneity of the compartments with respect to the CA distribution, a CA flux that is proportional to the concentration gradient between compartments, a negligible contribution from diffusion of CA from other voxels and a time invariance of the compartment volumes and permeability coefficients. Further compartmentalization of the CA within the extravascular extracellular space is ignored. Finally the water exchange between compartments is assumed to be fast so that a single relaxation time constant T_1 can be measured for the tissue, although the CA is compartmentalized. The Tofts and Kermode model [41] fails in areas where contrast extraction from the vasculature is extensive (flow limited case) or negligible, such as in normal brain tissue.

5.3. Steady state techniques

The so called steady state approaches for CBV measurement rely on the signal or relaxation rate change induced by a CA after having reached a homogeneous distribution and stable concentration in the intravascular compartment [45, 46]. Since CAs with a long blood half life and high relaxivity or a comparatively high CA dose is needed, they are only used in the research setting.

T_1 [47, 48], T_2 [49] or T_2^* weighted acquisitions are performed before and after injection of the CA, to determine the signal difference ΔS or the relaxation rate change ΔR_1, ΔR_2 or ΔR_2^* in the brain tissue before and after injection of a CA. To quantify the CBV with steady state techniques, measurement of the signal change, relaxation rate change or susceptibility difference induced by the CA in the blood compartment is needed. Although limited by the partial volume effect, this information can be obtained from a vascular ROI to avoid blood sampling.

Quantitative CBV is calculated as the ratio of the signal or relaxation rate changes induced by the CA in tissue and blood: CBV = $\Delta S_{tissue}/ \Delta S_{blood}$ [47, 48] or CBV = $\Delta R_{i\,tissue}/ \Delta R_{i\,blood}$ with i = 1,2 [50].

Other studies [51, 52] have exploited the changes in R_2^* [29]. The CBV quantification by the steady state ΔR_2^* method is based on a simplified geometric model of the brain microvasculature and the approximation of quasi static water protons. The compartmentalization of CAs, such as ultrasmall superparamagnetic nanoparticles of iron oxide (USPIO) characterized by a high magnetic susceptibility, within the randomly oriented capillary network of the brain results in localized microscopic field inhomogeneities in the tissue in which water protons diffuse, inducing a loss of transverse phase coherence with T_2^* signal loss in the perivascular space. The component of the magnetic field B(r) which is parallel to B_0 is inversely proportional to the square of the distance r form the vessel $B(r) \propto \Delta M (R/r)^2 \sin^2(\Theta)$ and it is a function of the magnetization difference ΔM between the intra- and extravascular compartment induced by the compartmentalized CA, the vessel radius R and the angle Θ between the direction of the main magnetic field B_0 and the axis of the vessel (Fig. 3). A quasi static water proton diffusion regime assumes that the mean diffusion length of the extravascular water proton d = $(D\, TE)^{1/2}$ is short with respect to the vessel radius R. In this case, the water protons situated at different distances r from the vessel experience different magnetic field strengths B(r) and therefore diphase at different rates.

The proportionality factor between the vascular volume fraction and relaxation rate difference ΔR_2^* induced by the presence of the CA depends on the intra-extravascular susceptibility difference $\Delta\chi$. Monte Carlo simulations show good agreement with in vivo results [45, 53]. However $\Delta\chi$ has to be measured from blood samples and is sensitive to differences in hematocrit and oxygenation between the sampled blood and the microvasculature [54, 55].

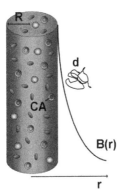

Figure 3. The ΔR_2^* method for CBV measurement models the capillary as an infinitely long and homogeneous cylinder containing the CA. The magnetic field gradient around the cylinder is a function of the cylinder radius R, of the magnetization difference between the intra- and extravascular compartment, of the cylinder orientation in the main homogeneous magnetic field B_0 and of the distance from the cylinder r. The diffusion regime is said to be quasi static when the mean water proton diffusion length d is short with respect to R, in such a way that the water protons in the vicinity of the cylinder dephase at a faster rate than those situated further away.

The CBV fraction is obtained in the following way [56]:

$$CBV = \frac{3}{4\pi} \frac{1}{\gamma \Delta X B_0} \Delta R_2^*$$

where γ is the gyromagnetic ratio and B_0 is the static magnetic field strength.

The ratio $\Delta R_2^*/\Delta R_2$ is dependent on the vessel size [45, 57]. ΔR_2 is sensitive primarily to small vessels, while ΔR_2^* is influenced by a broader range of vessel sizes. By measuring $\Delta R_2^*/\Delta R_2$ using gradient echo and spin echo sequences, and the water diffusion coefficient D, it is possible to estimate the VSI: VSI = 0.424 $(D/\gamma \Delta \chi B_0)^{1/2}(\Delta R_2^*/\Delta R_2)^{3/2}$.

5.4. Vascular space occupancy technique

The vascular space occupancy (VASO) technique [58] is a T_1 weighted technique that uses an inversion recovery sequence with timing parameters optimized to suppress the blood signal, while the extravascular tissue gives rise to a signal, which is not at its equilibrium value. For functional MRI, images are acquired during task performance (regional CBV change) and under rest conditions. It is assumed that the sum of intravascular and extravascular magnetization in a voxel is equal in the rest and in the activated condition and consequently a CBV change would inversely affect the extravascular magnetization. The signal difference between the rest and the activated condition is proportional to the CBV change. A signal decrease of about 0.7% has been detected under task performance consistent with a vasodilation [58]}.

In a quantitative version of this approach [59], the absolute CBV can be determined using the T_1 shortening effect of a CA. The signal before CA injection S_{pre} is only of extravascular origin since the blood signal is suppressed by the inversion recovery sequence using an appropriate inversion time T_{inv}: $S_{pre} = S_{ev}$ where S_{ev} is the extravascular signal. After CA injection, the T_{inv} is sufficiently long to allow full relaxation of the blood water magnetization to thermodynamic equilibrium, and the post-contrast signal S_{post} is given by: $S_{post} = S_{ev} + S_{0\,iv}$ where $S_{0\,iv}$ is the blood signal corresponding to the thermodynamic equilibrium magnetization of the blood compartment. The signals in the difference image are proportional to the blood volume since the extravascular tissue cancels out: $S_{post} - S_{pre} = S_{0\,iv}$.

This method is similar to the steady state T_1 weighted approach except that the equilibrium signal of the blood is acquired directly. For CBV quantification, the resulting blood signal in the difference image is normalized by the signal corresponding to the thermodynamic equilibrium magnetization of the total tissue (intra- + extravascular compartment). The normalization factor is obtained from a ROI containing cerebrospinal fluid on a reference image with sufficiently long acquisition times or from a small ROI containing mainly blood on the postcontrast image.

In humans, mean CBV of 1.4 and 5.5 ml/100 g have been measured with this technique for white matter and cortical gray matter, respectively [59].

The main difficulty encountered with this technique is that the repetition time (TR = 6 s) used is relatively long and therefore the blood T_1 has to be known precisely in order to determine the blood nulling inversion time ($T_{inv} \approx 1s$, depending on the field strength). A slightly inappropriate T_{inv}, reduced inversion efficiency or a change in blood T_1 (e.g. with hematocrit or oxygenation) results in a non negligible negative or positive blood signal before CA injection leading to a misestimation of the CBV in the difference image. Moreover, due to a relatively long T_{inv}, the water exchange between intra- and extravascular compartment will have a large effect. Finally, if the normalization factor is obtained from a vascular ROI affected by a partial volume effect, the CBV might be overestimated.

5.5. The rapid steady state T_1 technique

The Rapid Steady State T_1 (RSST$_1$) technique [60] is a quantitative T_1 weighted MRI technique for cerebral BVf mapping combining features of dynamic and steady state methods. Like the previously described methods it is based on a two-compartment model of the brain (intra- and extravascular) and necessitates the intravenous injection of a CA. It uses an inversion recovery (IR) prepared MRI sequence, but, in contrast to the VASO technique, a short repetition time (TR < 1 s). For such a short TR a dynamic equilibrium of the longitudinal magnetization M_z installs in which slowly relaxing magnetization never reaches its thermodynamic equilibrium value. In addition, for tissues with $T_1 > 1$ s, such as blood without CA and extravascular tissue, M_z crosses the null line at almost the same inversion time T_{inv} (Figure 4 a). The images are acquired using a fast low flip angle gradient echo imaging sequence FLASH [61, 62] and making sure the central k-space line is acquired when the longitudinal magnetization component crosses the null line (Figure 4 b). The signal evolution during this pulse sequence can be modeled [63]. Equation 4 is an approximation for the longitudinal magnetization M_z for low flip angles α, when dynamic equilibrium has installed:

$$\frac{M_z\left(T_{inv},TR,T_1\right)}{M_0} = 1 - \frac{2\exp\left(-\dfrac{T_{inv}}{T_1}\right)}{1+\exp\left(-\dfrac{TR}{T_1}\right)} \tag{4}$$

where M_0 is the longitudinal magnetization at thermodynamic equilibrium and TR the repetition time between two inversion pulses. Suppression of the longitudinal tissue magnetization can be achieved for

$$T_{inv}(TR,T_1) = T_1\ln 2 - T_1\ln\left[1+\exp\left(-\frac{TR}{T_1}\right)\right].$$

Figure 4 c shows M_z in function of T_1 for different T_{inv} and TR = 750 ms.

Using a TR/T_{inv} couple such as 750 ms/325 ms or 500 ms/225 ms, the IR-FLASH sequence acts like a T_1 low pass filter suppressing extravascular signals having high T_1 values and selectively acquiring the intravascular signal in the presence of a CA. In particular, a blood signal at thermodynamic equilibrium is acquired when the blood T_1 is below a critical value $T_{1blood} \approx T_{inv}/5$ after CA injection (Figure 4 a), reflecting the quantity of intravascular water protons. To quantify the BVf, the acquired blood signal S is normalized to the thermodynamic equilibrium (proton density weighted) signal of the intra- plus extravascular tissue water S_0 [60] obtained in an acquisition with sufficiently long TR. To eliminate residual signal from extravascular compartments, such as from white matter that has lower T_1, in particular at low magnetic field strength, the average signal acquired before CA injection $\{S_{pre}\}$ is subtracted before normalization. The normalized vascular signal S_{norm} is then given by

$$S_{norm\,i} = \left(S_i - \langle S_{pre}\rangle\right)/S_0$$

where S is the RSST$_1$-signal and i denotes the time frame.

A plot of S_{norm} over time during and after CA injection is shown in Figure 5. For a low CA dose, the signal time course resembles the one in Fig 2 as long as the signal is dependent on the CA concentration in blood. However, when $T_{1blood} \leq T_{inv}/5$ during the first pass the signal is saturated and its amplitude equals the CBV fraction. For a higher CA dose, T_{1blood} can be sufficiently low for the second pass or for a longer time interval. Note that in contrast to steady state techniques, the CA concentration does not need to be in a steady state to result in a steady state signal. The name of the technique "rapid steady state" was chosen to describe the dynamic equilibrium of the signal when it becomes independent of the CA concentration, not the contrast agent concentration in blood itself.

In this way the RSST$_1$ technique bypasses the need for conversion of the signal intensity change into relaxation rate change and the assumption of proportionality between the latter and CA concentration. The concomitant T_2 effect of the CA is minimized by using acquisitions with short TE.

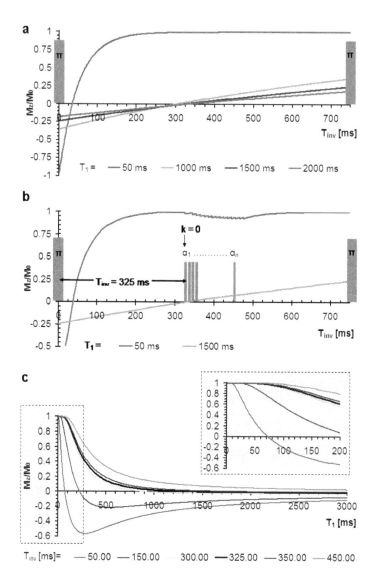

Figure 4. a: The longitudinal magnetization component M_z in an IR sequence with 750 ms repetition time is plotted after dynamic equilibrium has installed. M_z is suppressed and crosses the zero line at almost the same T_{inv} for tissues with long T_1, while for the same T_{inv} M_z is at thermodynamic equilibrium for tissues with short T_1 such as blood in presence of the CA. π = nonselective inversion pulse. b: The FLASH module acquires the image (and in particular the k = 0 line) when M_z of tissues with long T_1 crosses the zero-line and blood magnetization is fully relaxed (due to the T_1 shortening effect of a vascular CA). Here a center-out acquisition scheme is illustrated. α = low flip angle pulse. c: Equation 4 is plotted as a function of T_1 for several T_{inv} and TR = 750 ms. For T_{inv} = 325 ms M_z is suppressed for all $T_1 \geq 1$ s while it relaxes to thermodynamic equilibrium for $T_1 \leq 65$ ms as shown in the zoom.

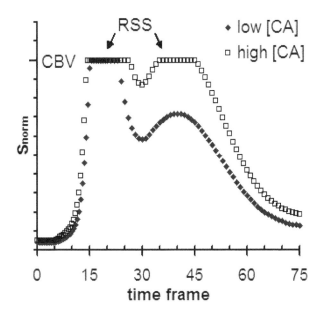

Figure 5. Plot of S_{norm} over time. At a particular CA concentration [CA] during first and sometimes also during the second pass or longer, S_{norm} does not depend on the [CA] any more but reaches a rapid steady state (RSS) value, corresponding to the BVf.

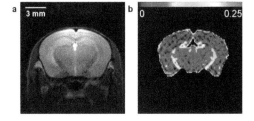

Figure 6. a: Coronal MRI image of a mouse brain showing structural details. b: Corresponding S_{norm} map showing an average cerebral BVf of 0.02 ± 0.004 and demonstrating CA accumulation in the cerebrospinal fluid leading to overestimation of the CBV in periventricular structures.

The $RSST_1$ technique was developed with CAs that remain confined to the vascular space during the measurement such as the clinically approved small molecular size CA Gd-DOTA from Guerbet Laboraories in the presence of an intact blood brain barrier (BBB) [60]. CAs with more convenient properties are available for preclinical applications. The experimental CA P760 from Guerbet Laboratories is an intermediate molecular size CA with higher relaxivities and higher intravascular restriction (molecular weight 5.29 kDa versus 0.55 kDa, mean diameter 2.8 nm versus 0.9 nm, longitudinal relaxivity $r_1 = 17.2$ mM^{-1}s^{-1} versus 2.9 mM^{-1}s^{-1}, transverse relaxivity $r_2 = 27.1$ mM^{-1}s^{-1} versus 4.8 mM^{-1}s^{-1} at 2.35 T, [64]). A rapid steady state of at least 30 s can be obtained starting at a dose of 0.15 mmol/kg Gd-DOTA and 0.035 mmol/kg P760 at 2.35T. However, quantitative CBV maps were obtained in healthy rats with P760 at a dose of 0.1 mmol/kg and with Gd-DOTA at a dose of 0.2 to 0.3 mmol/kg. These CA doses lead to a RSS interval of up to 5 minutes that can be used for increasing the SNR, the in-plane resolution or the number of slices. Even longer RSS intervals were obtained using a continuous infusion of these CA [60]. Quantitative CBV maps were also obtained in mice at 4.7T [65]. Due to faster hemodynamics in mice and reduced relaxivities of Gd-DOTA at higher magnetic field strength, an intravenous 0.7 mmol/kg dose was used. To lengthen the RSS, the intraperitoneal administration route has been employed in mice using a 6 mmol/kg dose which was well tolerated and lead to a RSS interval of about 30 minutes starting 15 minutes after injection. Quantitatively equivalent CBV measures were obtained using the intravenous and intraperitoneal routes on the same mice. A representative coronal CBV fraction map of a healthy mouse is shown in Figure 6. In studies performed repeatedly (once per month) in the same mice the cerebral BVf was well correlated between time points (Spearman r = 0.94, P-value = 0.017), with an intraindividual variability of the BVf measure in the caudate putamen of 0.018 to 0.024 (mean ± standard deviation: 0.022 ± 0.003) demonstrating the reproducibility of the CBV quantification. Intraperitoneal CA administration has the advantage of being less invasive with a lower risk for emboli and hypervolemia than intravenous administration. However, the CBV in cerebral regions close to ventricles might be overestimated due to CA arrival from the cerebrospinal fluid in which the CA accumulates.

The sensitivity of the RSST$_1$ technique to detect CBV changes has been assessed. In rats, the measurement has been repeated under different capnia conditions [60]. Hypercapnia is induced by breathing elevated levels of carbon dioxide and results in vasodilation. In mice the vasodilator acetazolamide has been injected during the long vascular RSS interval obtained after intraperitoneal Gd-DOTA injection [65]. In both experiments, the technique has been found to be sensitive to the BVf change (Figure 7) and the degree of change was comparable with published values using different techniques [66-68].

The quantification of tumor angiogenesis is complicated by the leakiness of the vessels for these CA leading to an overestimation of the CBV in the presence of CA leakage when using

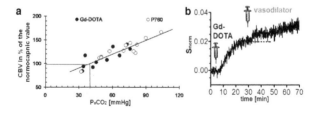

Figure 7. a: A hypercapnia experiment demonstrates CBV increase in healthy rats. b: In healthy mice, the S$_{norm}$ signal during the RSS increases shortly after intraperitoneal injection of the vasodilator acetazolamide.

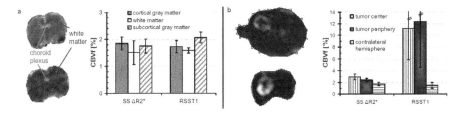

Figure 8.

a T_1 weighted technique. Two strategies are possible: I) Injection of CAs that remain confined to the vasculature despite hyperpermeable endothelium, and II) monitoring the CA accumulation in tumor tissue to be analyzed using an appropriate two compartment model.

USPIO such as AMI 227 (Sinerem, Guerbet Laboratories, Combidex, AMAG Pharmaceuticals) are widely used for their blood pool properties. They have also been used to quantify the blood volume fraction in malignant tumors in preclinical studies [69-72]. AMI 227 has a r^2 relaxivity in the order of 100 mM^{-1}s^{-1} and is mainly used in T^2 or T^{2*} weighted acquisitions. The r1 relaxivity of AMI 227 (r^1 = 5.4 mM^{-1}s^{-1} at 2.35T) together with its blood pool property, makes it an attractive CA for a T^1 weighted technique. Sequences with ultrashort echo time (TE) need to be used to exploit the T^1 effect. Acquisition schemes starting at the center of k-space such as radial or spiral acquisitions achieve short TE. A 3D projection reconstruction acquisition mode with a TE = 0.7 ms, was used at 2.35T to map the CBV with the RSST^1 technique using 0.2 mmol/kg AMI 227 in healthy and tumor bearing rats [73]. The post injection acquisition lasted 24 minutes, for which a steady state CA concentration in blood was assumed. The CBV measurement was compared with a steady state ΔR^{2*} technique in the same animals (Figure 8 a). After correction for transverse relaxation effects, both acquisition techniques yielded comparable results in healthy rat brain and a C6 glioma model. However, in a RG2 glioma model, the RSST1 technique yielded high tumor BVf while in the same ROIs the steady state ΔR^{2*} technique yielded BVfs that were significantly lower than in healthy or contralateral tissue (Figure 8 b). Such a discrepancy can only be explained by loss of CA compartmentalization, which results in underestimation of the BVf with T^{2*} weighted techniques while T1 weighted acquisitions tend to overestimate the BVf. There is also evidence for AMI 227 extravasation in the RG2 tumor model in results published by other authors [69].

In the search for intravascular CA with high r_1 relaxivity for tumor BVf quantification, good results were obtained with a novel preclinical CA based on a modified cyclodextrin [74] in a C6 tumor model [75]. This paramagnetic CA is an inclusion complex of Gd^{3+} with per-(3,6-anhydro)-α-cyclodextrin. It has a molecular weight of 1464 Dalton and the shape of a flat disc. The relaxivities of Gd-ACX decrease with increased concentration, but at a 1.5 mM concentration in normal saline at 2.35T relaxivities are still r_1 = 8.6 s^{-1}mM^{-1} and r_2 = 10.4 s^{-1}mM^{-1} about twice as high as for Gd-DOTA [64]. The biodistribution of Gd-ACX (0.05 mmol/kg) and the CBVf were studied using T_1 weighted imaging and the RSST$_1$ technique at 2.35T in healthy and C6 tumor bearing Wistar rats 20 and 21 days after implantation, and compared to

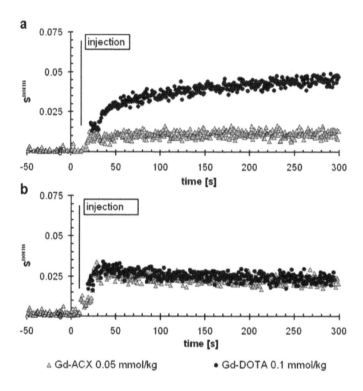

Figure 9. S_{norm} versus time curves after Gd-ACX and Gd-DOTA injection in C6 glioma tissue (a) and contralateral brain tissue (b). There is no evidence of Gd-ACX extravasation during the first 5 minutes after injection enabling BVf quantification in presence of vascular endothelium permeable to Gd-DOTA.

quantitative CBVf maps and the regional signal enhancement obtained after injection of Gd-DOTA. After Gd-ACX injection, the signal enhancement appears immediately in large vessels, but not in the tumor, while injection of Gd-DOTA reveals disruption of the BBB since an extensive signal enhancement is observed inside the tumor area. Representative signal versus time plots from one rat obtained by the $RSST_1$ method in the tumor periphery and in contralateral brain tissue are shown in Fig. 9 a and b respectively. After Gd-ACX injection, S_{norm} remains constant for about 5 min, while after Gd-DOTA injection the signal in tumor tissue increases continuously, reflecting CA accumulation due to a BBB leakage for this CA. Identical signal behavior in cerebral tissue contralateral to the tumor after injection of Gd-ACX and Gd-DOTA is observed (Figure 9 b). The constant signal enhancement obtained with the $RSST_1$ technique during the first five minutes confirms the absence of immediate Gd-ACX Extravasation from tumor vasculature allowing quantification of the tumor BVf using Gd-ACX in presence of vascular permeability to Gd-DOTA. However, the modest thermodynamic stability of Gd-ACX will limit its use to preclinical studies. For clinical applications, tumor angiogenesis needs to be assessed with clinically approved low molecular weight CA such as Gd-DOTA despite CA leakage.

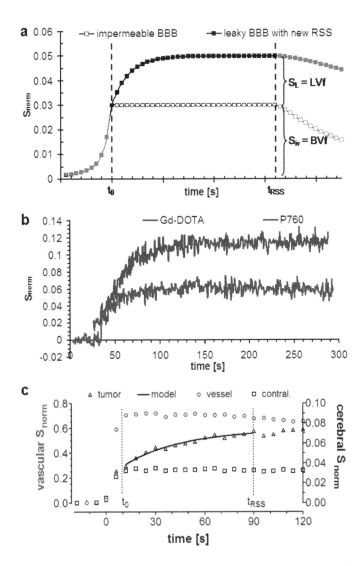

Figure 10. A model of the signal evolution during CA arrival and distribution in the tissue for two ROIs. The lower plot represents the signal in a RSS from a ROI, in which the CA is confined to the blood pool. The upper plot displays the idealized shape of a leakage profile during the vascular RSS time window $[t_0, t_{RSS}]$ attaining a new RSS at a signal amplitude corresponding to the sum of BVf and LVf. CA = contrast agent, RSS = rapid steady state, ROI = region of interest, BVf = blood volume fraction, LVf = leakage volume fraction. b: Typical leakage profiles for a low (Gd-DOTA) and intermediate molecular size (P760) CA in a RG2 tumor model demonstrating that the vascular permeability and the total distribution volume is lower for the larger CA. c: Modeled leakage profile for Gd-DOTA in a C6 tumor model (right axis) along with RSS profiles for signal from a large vessel (left axis) and contralateral brain tissue (right axis) defining the time window $[t_0, t_{RSS}]$ for leakage monitoring.

Unlike steady state techniques and similar to DCE-MRI, the high temporal resolution of the $RSST_1$ technique enables monitoring of dynamic signal changes as illustrated in Figure 5.. Due to the use of high relaxivity CA or high doses in preclinical studies, the vascular RSS is maintained over several minutes beyond the first pass. In tissues with permeable vasculature the CA extravasates leading to a continuous signal increase. If the time window for which the vascular signal corresponds to the BVf is known, the CA accumulation in tissue with permeable vasculature can be modeled. The model assumes two compartments accessible to the CA: the blood and the extravascular leakage compartment. The remaining compartments, not attained by the CA, maintain a high T_1 value and do not lead to significant signal. The S_{norm} signal reaches a RSS when the CA reaches a uniform concentration in the distribution compartment leading to a sufficiently low T_1. As illustrated in Figure "10 a, in case of CA leakage the signal time course approaches an asymptote. The maximum signal enhancement is then composed of the BVf and the leakage volume fraction (LVf). The S_{norm} signal is modeled as:

$$S_{model}(t) = S_{iv} + S_L \left\{ 1 - \exp\left[-\kappa(t - t_0)\right] \right\} \tag{5}$$

where t_0 is the beginning of the RSS time interval which can be obtained from a large vascular structure or brain tissue with intact BBB. The BVf is estimated as S_{iv}, i.e. S_{model} in the beginning of the signal RSS. S_L is the proton density weighted signal of the extravascular leakage compartment approximating the local extravascular distribution volume fraction (i.e. the LVf) of the CA. κ is a parameter related to the leakage rate. The CA leakage is assumed to be permeability limited [41]. Setting BVf = S_{iv} also assumes negligible CA extravasation in the beginning of the first pass of the CA bolus. CA backflow from the extravascular leakage compartment into the blood is not taken into account. A comparison of leakage signal profiles for two CA with different molecular weight in the same tumor tissue are shown in Figure 10 b, showing that the larger CA has a slower leakage rate and a lower distribution volume. Using Gd-DOTA, analysis of the leakage profile can therefore give valuable information about the vascular permeability which is spatially and temporally heterogenous in malignant tumors. Figure 10 c shows how the RSS time window can be determined from tissue containing impermeable vasculature in order to limit the fitting procedure to this time interval. This is not equivalent to the definition of an AIF, since the actual signal intensity is not of importance.

The described methodological development of the $RSST_1$ technique was carried out at magnetic field strengths above 2.35T necessitating injection of high CA doses in order to compensate for the decreasing CA relaxivity with higher field strength and to achieve long vascular RSS intervals for signal averaging to overcome the low SNR in small animal imaging. In the clinical setting, the method is not only limited to Gd-DOTA-like CA, but also to low doses. In routine imaging a dose of 0.1 mmol/kg is administered, but a double or triple dose has been shown to result in higher sensitivity in particular applications. However, gadolinium based CA can result in serious complications such as nephritic systemic fibrosis in susceptible patients, it is therefore cautious to limit the administered dose to a minimum.

A pilot experiment on a 3T Philips Achieva research MRI scanner showed that CBV quantification with the $RSST_1$ technique in the primate (macaque) brain is feasible with a 0.2 mmol/kg

Gd-DOTA dose at this field strength. In order to reduce the Gd-DOTA dose, the $RSST_1$ technique has been implemented on a clinical 1.5T Philips Achieva scanner where it was integrated in the routine imaging protocol for follow up studies of neurooncological patients. The routine imaging protocol necessitated Gd-DOTA administration to look for pathological contrast enhancement on T_1 weighted images, but did not include perfusion imaging techniques. A number of 120 $RSST_1$ acquisitions (TR/T_{inv} = 750 ms/315 ms, matrix 64 x 55, flip angle 10º, inter-echo repetition time 4 ms, TE = 1.2 ms) were acquired over 90 s before, during and after CA injection using an automatic injector with an injection rate of 6 ml/s. These acquisitions were normalized to the proton density acquisition acquired before injection using the same sequence without inversion pulse and a TR of 10 s (number of averages = 3). Patients were injected with either 15 ml (= 7.5 mmol) or 30 ml (15 mmol) Gd-DOTA according to their reported or estimated weight as is often done in clinical routine, but weighted after completed examination in order to determine the administered dose precisely. In the feasibility studies, the imaging plane was chosen to include large vessels such as the basilar artery or branches of the circle of Willis and a large dural venous sinus to study the vascular signal with minimal partial volume effect. An example of the S_{norm}-signal profile is shown in Figure 11. It can be observed that during the first pass of the CA S_{norm} reaches a value of 1 (one) corresponding to 100% blood when the voxel is placed within the vessel without partial volume effect. Consequently, the S_{norm} amplitude in brain tissue during the first pass reflects the CBV fraction. At 1.5T, a Gd-DOTA dose of 0.13 mmol/kg is necessary for reliable quantitative CBV fraction mapping. Below this dose, a sufficiently high CA concentration in the brain vasculature is only achieved for patients with a relatively low body mass index. The determined optimum dose is 30% higher than the recommended Gd-DOTA dose but still approved and often used in clinical practice. A RSS interval limited to the first pass of the CA has the following advantages: First, extravasation from hyperpermeable vasculature is minimized. When significant CA extravasation occurs, it can be detected as an increasing instead of a constant signal, and algorithms for leakage correction can be applied. Second, hemodynamic information can be derived. Like the mean transit time, the duration of the RSS during the first pass is related to the blood flow, but similar to first pass perfusion techniques it is also determined by the CA injection rate, dispersion and the BVf. As with first pass perfusion techniques the RSS duration relative to a reference region might still have diagnostic value.

6. What are the confounding effects?

To evaluate the accuracy of the $RSST_1$ technique confounding effects need to be taken into consideration. For example, the signal attenuation due to transverse relaxation has been minimized by using short TE. When T_2^* attenuation was significant as with AMI 227, the blood T_2^* after injection has been measured to estimate and correct for this effect.

The $RSST_1$ technique is not sensitive to blood flow effects that often affect quantification in dynamic perfusion techniques. First, the inversion pulse is not slice selective, inverting all proton spins whether they are stationary, mobile, in the imaging plane or not. Second, when the blood T_1 is sufficiently low after CA injection, the blood flowing into the imaging plane

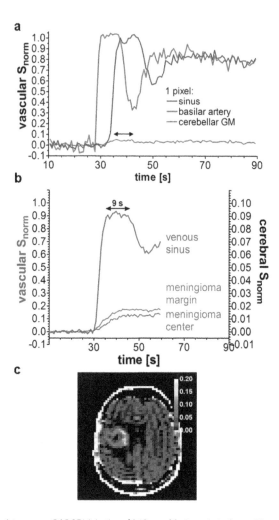

Figure 11. a: After an intravenous Gd-DOTA injection of 0.13 mmol/kg in patients, S_{norm} = 1 is attained during the first pass in large vascular structures without partial volume effect. The S_{norm} amplitude in brain tissue during the first pass (arrow) therefore corresponds to the BVf. S_{norm} = 0.04 in the cerebellar gray matter (GM) voxel. b: While the vascular signal is in a RSS for about 9 s in this patient, a typical CA leakage profile is observed in the meningioma tissue. c: S_{norm} map of a patient with glioblastoma. No leakage correction was applied and the BVf of 8 to 10% in the tumor border might be overestimated if significant CA leakage occurred during the first pass.

between the excitation pulse and the readout arrives with a magnetization at thermal equilibrium such as the blood flowing out of the imaging plane.

However, the RSST$_1$ technique seeks to selectively acquire signal from water molecules that are in contact with the CA. The mobility of water molecules and their exchange across the vessel wall might affect the CBV quantification. For example, water molecules that relax with a short T_1 because they were in contact with the CA in the vascular compartment, but happen to exchange to the extravascular compartment during the inversion time, will reduce the extravascular T_1. This might lead to a signal contribution from the extravascular compartment and therefore to a CBV overestimation. The $RSST_1$ technique is based on a two compartment model and assumes negligible water exchange between these compartments. Whether the exchange regime is fast or slow depends on the water exchange rate and on the difference between the longitudinal relaxation rates of the intravascular and extravascular compartment. An intracapillary residence time of 500 to 650 ms has been reported for healthy brain tissue [76] leading to a transendothelial exchange rate in the order of 2 s^{-1} which is slow compared to the difference of the longitudinal relaxation rates between the two compartments which is in the order of 20 s^{-1} at the peak CA concentration. The exchange effect on the CBV measure was evaluated using the model described in Moran and Prato [77] and showed an overestimation of 10 -12% for a T_{inv} of 325 ms and an assumed vascular T_1 of 50 ms during the RSS. The water exchange effect is more pronounced for higher CA agent doses or relaxivities such as used in preclinical studies. It can be reduced by shortening T_{inv}, allowing the compartments less time to exchange water across the vascular boundary. For example, with the couple of parameters TR = 500 ms and Tinv = 225 ms, the overestimation would be reduced to less than 4% for a vascular T_1 of 45 ms.

Strictly speaking, the blood as well as the extravascular compartment are multi compartment systems. The CA molecules do not enter the cells. However, the blood can be considered as a single compartment because even in the presence of CA molecules in plasma the intra-extracellular difference of the longitudinal relaxation rates is still one order of magnitude lower than the water exchange rate between erythrocytes and plasma ($\tau_{exch}^{-1} \approx 125$ s^{-1}). In this fast exchange limit, the intracellular water is affected by the presence of the CA, and it is the CBV that is measured and not the plasma volume. It is therefore not necessary to correct for the regional hematocrit.

7. How to validate a quantitative blood volume measure?

When developing new acquisition or analysis techniques the validity of their assumptions and their limits need to be assessed using reference methods ideally on the same brain. This implies either using a MRI technique that does not rely on the same principle or on the same assumptions or a technique that has a different signal origin. Experimental and physiologic conditions need to be kept as similar as possible, which is not straightforward when the subject or animal needs to be moved from one scanner to another or when the measurements are a long time interval apart or relay on CAs with different properties. In particular, comparisons between in vivo and ex vivo techniques have to be interpreted with caution since the "physiologic" conditions are not alike. Nevertheless, histological validation is still the gold standard. When evaluating angiogenesis by histology, surrogate markers such as microvascular density or vascular area density are often used because they can be directly quantified from two-dimensional histological sections. The vascular volume density comes closest to the BVf but necessitates a stereological analysis of vascular morphometric data.

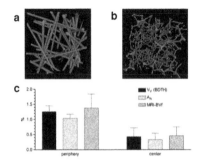

Figure 12. Validation of the C6 tumor BVf measured with Gd-ACX and the $RSST_1$ technique. a and b: Numerical models used to evaluate the stereological approach: cylinder model (a) and cortical mouse vasculature (b). The stereological analysis of vascular morphometry confirms the tumor BVf measured by MRI (c).

To validate the tumor BVf obtained with Gd-ACX by MRI, the vascular volume density was calculated as $V_v = \pi\{d\}^2 L_v/4$ where $\{d\}$ is the mean vessel diameter and L_v is the vascular length density obtained using a stereological analysis technique proposed by Adair [78]. For quantitative analysis of the microvasculature, 20 approximately equally spaced sections of 10 μm thickness were cut from the same location as the MR image (2 mm thickness). The collagen IV component of the vascular endothelium was stained using a fluorescent marker and the intravitally injected Hoechst dye was used to mark vessels which were perfused at the moment of injection. The tissue sections were digitized using a 10× magnification. ImageJ was used for segmentation and vascular morphometry. The stereological technique approximates the vessel sections as elliptical profiles of vessels modeled as randomly oriented straight cylinders. The vessel orientation was determined from the ratio of major and minor ellipse axes in order to derive L_v as described in [78]. However, no gold standard parameter exists that defines the vessels diameter from an irregularly shaped vessel cross section. Therefore, four morphologic parameters were analyzed for their potential utility as descriptors for the vessel diameter: the radius of the inscribed circle, the minor axis of the fitted ellipses, the small side of the bounding box and the breadth. They were evaluated on a simulated idealized cylinder model and on mouse cortical vasculature obtained from two-photon microscopy data (Figure "12). Only the breadth and the minor axis of ellipse yielded reliable and physiologically appropriate diameters. These numeric data was also used to evaluate the minimum number of sections necessary to reliably quantify stereologic parameters such as the L_v. After these optimizations the stereological analysis was applied to healthy rat brain and C6 tumor tissue and yielded vascular volume densities similar to the BVf measured by MRI with Gd-ACX. However, it was shown that only half of the tumor vessels detectable by histology were functional (perfused) vessels that contribute to the BVf measurement by MRI.

In opposite to the RG2 glioma model, the rat C6-glioma model has microvasculature permeable to Gd-DOTA but not to superparamagnetic iron-oxide nanoparticles (USPIO) allowing validation of the BVf derived from the leakage signal time course of Gd-DOTA using a steady state ΔR_2^*-MRI method with an USPIO. Figure 13 a shows two BVf maps obtained with the two MRI techniques on the same animal. Despite different spatial resolution both BVf maps reflect almost the same values and heterogeneity in the tumor. The tumor BVf and the contralateral cerebral BVf of 0.034 ± 0.005 and 0.026 ± 0.004, respectively, were confirmed, in the same rats, by ΔR_2^*-MRI (0.036 ± 0.003 and 0.027 ± 0.002) and also by immunohistochemical staining (anti-collagen type IV) of perfused vessels (0.036 ± 0.003 and 0.025 ± 0.004) labeled with intravitally injected Hoechst dye. Figure 13 b shows the correlation between the three techniques.

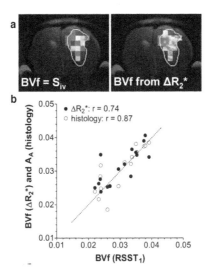

Figure 13. Validation of the BVf obtained in a C6 tumor with the $RSST_1$ technique by modeling the leakage signal profile of Gd-DOTA a: Tumor BVf maps obtained with the $RSST_1$ and a steady state ΔR_2^* technique with an USPIO (MoldayION from BioPAL, Worcester, MA)as blood pool agent in the same animal show similar values and heterogeneity. b: Plot demonstrating the good correlation between BVf measured with the $RSST_1$ and the steady state ΔR_2^* and with the histological vascular area density.

However, in case of USPIO leakage such as is the case in RG2 tumor tissue, the loss of CA compartmentalization reduces the magnetization difference between intra- and extravascular compartment. The CBV then tends to be underestimated with ΔR_2^* methods.

8. What are the quantitative values of the regional blood volume in vivo?

CBV fraction values published for healthy rats are summarized in Table 1. They are in the range of 2 to 4% with regional and technique related differences. Using the $RSST_1$ technique with gadolinium based CA Gd-DOTA, P760 and Gd-ACX, regional CBV from 1.8 to 3.5% were measured in healthy rats (Table 1). When using AMI 227, a lower average CBV was measured (1.6 to 2.1%) and regional differences were less pronounced probably due to the transverse relaxation effect that was insufficiently corrected for and because of a lower spatial resolution. However, steady state ΔR_2^* measures in the same rats confirmed the low CBV (Figure 8). In C6 and RG2 tumor bearing rats, quantitative maps obtained with the $RSST_1$ technique revealed a significantly decreased contralateral CBV compared with healthy rats probably due to compression, edema, or inflammation [75], a finding also observed by other authors [71]. This shows that the vasculature in brain tissue contralateral to the tumor might not be representative of healthy brain vasculature as often assumed when reporting relative values. In a late stage C6 tumor model, a BVf of $0.98 \pm 0.34\%$ was measured in non necrotic tumor parts with the RSST1 technique and Gd-ACX, and confirmed by histology when care was taken to account for perfused vessels only.

MRI measurements in mice yield regional CBV fractions in the range of 1.7 to 2.7% including deep brain structures. Using intravital two-photon microscopy with an intravenously injected fluorescent marker, the BVf can be derived from the integrated fluorescence intensity [90]. The results in mouse brain cortex (2 to 2.4%) compare very well with the $RSST_1$ measures, however deeper structures are not measurable in vivo by two-photon microscopy presently limited to a depth of about 600 µm.

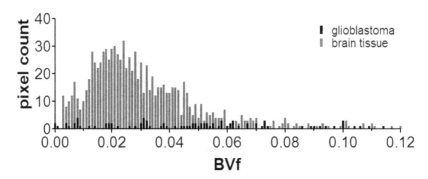

Figure 14.

In humans, BVf of 1.5 to 2.0% were measured in white matter, 3.5 to 4.5% in healthy appearing gray matter and values above 6% in glioblastoma margin. Figure 14 shows the BVf distribution in a healthy brain and in a glioblastoma after correction for CA leakage.

9. Conclusion

Direct quantitative mapping of the cerebral BVf is feasible with clinically approved contrast agents at a well tolerated dose during the first pass. The $RSST_1$ technique is powerful for the

ROI	CBV value	unit	technique	reference
corpus callosum	2.0 ± 0.3%	%	RSST$_1$ [b]	[60]
striatum	2.9 ± 0.6%	%	RSST$_1$ [b]	[60]
cortex	3.1 ± 0.8%	%	RSST$_1$ [b]	[60]
whole brain[a]	2.51	ml/100g	autoradiography[j]	[79]
whole brain[a]	2.96 ± 0.57	ml/100g	autoradiography[j]	[80]
whole brain[b]	2.77 ± 0.24	ml/100g	autoradiography[j]	[81]
whole brain	1.3 ± 0.1	ml/100g	autoradiography[j]	[82]
cortex	3.4	ml/100g	optical bolus tracking	[68]
whole brain[c]	2.40 ± 0.34	%	3D SS T$_1$ MRI	[48]
whole brain[c]	2.96 ± 0.82	%	3D SS T$_1$ MRI	[83]
whole brain[b]	3.14 ± 0.32	%	SST$_2$-MRI	[84]
cortex[b]	1.63 ± 0.18	ml/100g	SST$_1$-MRI	[85]
corpus callosum[b]	1.22 ± 0.25	ml/100g	SST$_1$-MRI	[85]
thalamus[b]	3.03 ± 0.36	ml/100g	SST$_1$-MRI	[85]
whole brain[b]	3.14 ± 0.32	%	SSΔR_2*-MRI	[84]
cortex[d]	4.3 ± 0.7	%	SSΔR_2*-MRI	[52]
striatum[e]	3.1 ± 0.7	ml/100g	SSΔR_2*-MRI	[86]
striatum[f]	2.2 ± 0.6	ml/100g	SSΔR_2*-MRI	[71]
cortex[a]	3.01 ± 0.43	%	SSΔR_2*-MRI	[51]
striatum[a]	2.94 ± 0.49	%	SSΔR_2*-MRI	[51]
cortex[a]	4.07	%	SSΔR_2*-MRI	[87]
striatum[a]	2.87	%	SSΔR_2*-MRI	[87]
whole brain	1.89 ± 0.39	%	morphometry[k]	[88]
whole brain without MV[g]	1.92 ± 0.32	ml/100g	SRQCT	[89]
whole brain with MV[g]	4.18 ± 1.06	ml/100g	SRQCT	[89]
cortex[g]	2.27	ml/100g	SRQCT	[89]
striatum[g]	2.01	ml/100g	SRQCT	[89]
striatum[h]	5.6	ml/100g	SRQCT	[89]

Reported values for the regional cerebral blood volume obtained with various imaging techniques. Decimal places and standard deviations are given as reported in the original work.

ROI = region of interest, MV = macroscopic vessels, CBV = cerebral blood volume, SST$_1$-MRI = steady state T$_1$-weighted magnetic resonance imaging, SSΔR_2*-MRI = steady state ΔR_2* magnetic resonance imaging, SRQCT = synchrotron radiation quantitative computed tomography

[a]rats anesthetized with halothane

[b]rats anesthetized with isoflurane

[c]rats anesthetized with intraperitoneal pentobarbital

[d]contralateral to C6 glioma, under moderate hypoxia, rats anesthetized with halothane

[e]rats anesthetized with intraperitoneal thiopental

[f]contralateral to C6 glioma, rats anesthetized with intraperitoneal thiopental

[g]anesthetized by intraperitoneal infusion of chloral hydrate

[h]contralateral to F98 glioma (n = 1)

[i]^{14}C-dextran labeled plasma and ^{99m}Tc labeled red blood cells

[j]^{125}I- labeled serum albumin and ^{55}Fe labeled red blood cells

[k]with stereo correction for slice thickness, contralateral to 9L tumor

Table 1. Regional cerebral blood volume (healthy regions) in normocapnic, normothermic, anesthetized rats.

clinical practice, because it can quantify the BVf simultaneously for vasculature with or without permeability to the contrast agent, without requiring the AIF and conversion of signal intensity into CA concentration. This technique will play an important role in treatment monitoring and clinical studies in particular for the evaluation of antiangiogenic agents.

Author details

Teodora-Adriana Perles-Barbacaru* and Hana Lahrech

*Address all correspondence to: teodora.perles-barbacaru@univ-amu.fr

Grenoble Institute of Neurosciences (GIN), French National Institute of Health and Medical Research (INSERM U) – University of Joseph Fourier (UJF) – French Atomic Energy Commission (CEA) – University Hospital of Grenoble (CHU), Bâtiment Edmond J. Safra, Chemin Fortuné Ferrini, La Tronche, France

References

[1] Aronen HJ, Gazit IE, Louis DN, Buchbinder BR, Pardo FS, Weisskoff RM, et al. Cerebral blood volume maps of gliomas: comparison with tumor grade and histologic findings. Radiology. 1994 Apr;191(1):41-51.

[2] Sugahara T, Korogi Y, Tomiguchi S, Shigematsu Y, Ikushima I, Kira T, et al. Posttherapeutic intraaxial brain tumor: the value of perfusion-sensitive contrast-enhanced MR imaging for differentiating tumor recurrence from nonneoplastic contrast-enhancing tissue. AJNR Am J Neuroradiol. 2000 May;21(5):901-9.

[3] Folkman J. New perspectives in clinical oncology from angiogenesis research. Eur J Cancer. 1996 Dec;32A(14):2534-9.

[4] Zama A, Tamura M, Inoue HK. Three-dimensional observations on microvascular growth in rat glioma using a vascular casting method. J Cancer Res Clin Oncol. 1991;117(5):396-402.

[5] Folkman J. The role of angiogenesis in tumor growth. Semin Cancer Biol. 1992 Apr; 3(2):65-71.

[6] Abdulrauf SI, Edvardsen K, Ho KL, Yang XY, Rock JP, Rosenblum ML. Vascular endothelial growth factor expression and vascular density as prognostic markers of survival in patients with low-grade astrocytoma. J Neurosurg. 1998 Mar;88(3):513-20.

[7] Assimakopoulou M, Sotiropoulou-Bonikou G, Maraziotis T, Papadakis N, Varakis I. Microvessel density in brain tumors. Anticancer Res. 1997 Nov-Dec;17(6D):4747-53.

[8] Brem S, Cotran R, Folkman J. Tumor angiogenesis: a quantitative method for histologic grading. J Natl Cancer Inst. 1972 Feb;48(2):347-56.

[9] Leon SP, Folkerth RD, Black PM. Microvessel density is a prognostic indicator for patients with astroglial brain tumors. Cancer. 1996 Jan 15;77(2):362-72.

[10] Revesz T, Scaravilli F, Coutinho L, Cockburn H, Sacares P, Thomas DG. Reliability of histological diagnosis including grading in gliomas biopsied by image-guided stereotactic technique. Brain. 1993 Aug;116 (Pt 4):781-93.

[11] Pardridge WM, Triguero D, Yang J, Cancilla PA. Comparison of in vitro and in vivo models of drug transcytosis through the blood-brain barrier. J Pharmacol Exp Ther. 1990 May;253(2):884-91.

[12] Duvernoy H, Delon S, Vannson JL. The vascularization of the human cerebellar cortex. Brain Res Bull. 1983 Oct;11(4):419-80.

[13] Herscovitch P, Raichle ME. What is the correct value for the brain--blood partition coefficient for water? J Cereb Blood Flow Metab. 1985 Mar;5(1):65-9.

[14] Taylor JS, Reddick WE. Evolution from empirical dynamic contrast-enhanced magnetic resonance imaging to pharmacokinetic MRI. Adv Drug Deliv Rev. 2000 Mar 15;41(1):91-110.

[15] Maeda M, Maley JE, Crosby DL, Quets JP, Zhu MW, Lee GJ, et al. Application of contrast agents in the evaluation of stroke: conventional MR and echo-planar MR imaging. J Magn Reson Imaging. 1997 Jan-Feb;7(1):23-8.

[16] Rosen BR. MR studies of perfusion in the brain. Current Practice in Radiology. Thrall, editor. Philadelphia, PA: Mosby Yearbook 1992.

[17] Rother J, Guckel F, Neff W, Schwartz A, Hennerici M. Assessment of regional cerebral blood volume in acute human stroke by use of single-slice dynamic susceptibility contrast-enhanced magnetic resonance imaging. Stroke. 1996 Jun;27(6):1088-93.

[18] Broom KA, Anthony DC, Blamire AM, Waters S, Styles P, Perry VH, et al. MRI reveals that early changes in cerebral blood volume precede blood-brain barrier breakdown and overt pathology in MS-like lesions in rat brain. J Cereb Blood Flow Metab. 2005 Feb;25(2):204-16.

[19] Sibson NR, Blamire AM, Perry VH, Gauldie J, Styles P, Anthony DC. TNF-alpha reduces cerebral blood volume and disrupts tissue homeostasis via an endothelin- and TNFR2-dependent pathway. Brain. 2002 Nov;125(Pt 11):2446-59.

[20] Looareesuwan S, Wilairatana P, Krishna S, Kendall B, Vannaphan S, Viravan C, et al. Magnetic resonance imaging of the brain in patients with cerebral malaria. Clin Infect Dis. 1995 Aug;21(2):300-9.

[21] Harris GJ, Lewis RF, Satlin A, English CD, Scott TM, Yurgelun-Todd DA, et al. Dynamic susceptibility contrast MRI of regional cerebral blood volume in Alzheimer's disease. Am J Psychiatry. 1996 May;153(5):721-4.

[22] Harris GJ, Lewis RF, Satlin A, English CD, Scott TM, Yurgelun-Todd DA, et al. Dynamic susceptibility contrast MR imaging of regional cerebral blood volume in Alzheimer disease: a promising alternative to nuclear medicine. AJNR Am J Neuroradiol. 1998 Oct;19(9):1727-32.

[23] Maas LC, Harris GJ, Satlin A, English CD, Lewis RF, Renshaw PF. Regional cerebral blood volume measured by dynamic susceptibility contrast MR imaging in Alzheimer's disease: a principal components analysis. J Magn Reson Imaging. 1997 Jan-Feb; 7(1):215-9.

[24] Ernst TM, Chang L, Witt MD, Aronow HA, Cornford ME, Walot I, et al. Cerebral toxoplasmosis and lymphoma in AIDS: perfusion MR imaging experience in 13 patients. Radiology. 1998 Sep;208(3):663-9.

[25] Tracey I, Hamberg LM, Guimaraes AR, Hunter G, Chang I, Navia BA, et al. Increased cerebral blood volume in HIV-positive patients detected by functional MRI. Neurology. 1998 Jun;50(6):1821-6.

[26] Garnett MR, Blamire AM, Corkill RG, Rajagopalan B, Young JD, Cadoux-Hudson TA, et al. Abnormal cerebral blood volume in regions of contused and normal appearing brain following traumatic brain injury using perfusion magnetic resonance imaging. J Neurotrauma. 2001 Jun;18(6):585-93.

[27] Cha S, Lu S, Johnson G, Knopp EA. Dynamic susceptibility contrast MR imaging: correlation of signal intensity changes with cerebral blood volume measurements. J Magn Reson Imaging. 2000 Feb;11(2):114-9.

[28] Dean BL, Lee C, Kirsch JE, Runge VM, Dempsey RM, Pettigrew LC. Cerebral hemodynamics and cerebral blood volume: MR assessment using gadolinium contrast agents and T1-weighted Turbo-FLASH imaging. AJNR Am J Neuroradiol. 1992 Jan-Feb;13(1):39-48.

[29] Villringer A, Rosen BR, Belliveau JW, Ackerman JL, Lauffer RB, Buxton RB, et al. Dynamic imaging with lanthanide chelates in normal brain: contrast due to magnetic susceptibility effects. Magn Reson Med. 1988 Feb;6(2):164-74.

[30] Kiselev VG. On the theoretical basis of perfusion measurements by dynamic susceptibility contrast MRI. Magn Reson Med. 2001 Dec;46(6):1113-22.

[31] Thompson HK, Jr., Starmer CF, Whalen RE, McIntosh HD. Indicator Transit Time Considered as a Gamma Variate. Circ Res. 1964 Jun;14:502-15.

[32] Meier P, Zierler KL. On the theory of the indicator-dilution method for measurement of blood flow and volume. J Appl Physiol. 1954 Jun;6(12):731-44.

[33] Calamante F, Gadian DG, Connelly A. Delay and dispersion effects in dynamic susceptibility contrast MRI: simulations using singular value decomposition. Magn Reson Med. 2000 Sep;44(3):466-73.

[34] Ostergaard L, Weisskoff RM, Chesler DA, Gyldensted C, Rosen BR. High resolution measurement of cerebral blood flow using intravascular tracer bolus passages. Part I: Mathematical approach and statistical analysis. Magn Reson Med. 1996 Nov;36(5): 715-25.

[35] Calamante F, Gadian DG, Connelly A. Quantification of perfusion using bolus tracking magnetic resonance imaging in stroke: assumptions, limitations, and potential implications for clinical use. Stroke. 2002 Apr;33(4):1146-51.

[36] Perthen JE, Calamante F, Gadian DG, Connelly A. Is quantification of bolus tracking MRI reliable without deconvolution? Magn Reson Med. 2002 Jan;47(1):61-7.

[37] Hacklander T, Hofer M, Reichenbach JR, Rascher K, Furst G, Modder U. Cerebral blood volume maps with dynamic contrast-enhanced T1-weighted FLASH imaging: normal values and preliminary clinical results. J Comput Assist Tomogr. 1996 Jul-Aug;20(4):532-9.

[38] Parker GJ, Suckling J, Tanner SF, Padhani AR, Revell PB, Husband JE, et al. Probing tumor microvascularity by measurement, analysis and display of contrast agent uptake kinetics. J Magn Reson Imaging. 1997 May-Jun;7(3):564-74.

[39] Flickinger FW, Allison JD, Sherry RM, Wright JC. Differentiation of benign from malignant breast masses by time-intensity evaluation of contrast enhanced MRI. Magn Reson Imaging. 1993;11(5):617-20.

[40] Tofts PS, Brix G, Buckley DL, Evelhoch JL, Henderson E, Knopp MV, et al. Estimating kinetic parameters from dynamic contrast-enhanced T(1)-weighted MRI of a diffusable tracer: standardized quantities and symbols. J Magn Reson Imaging. 1999 Sep;10(3):223-32.

[41] Tofts PS, Kermode AG. Measurement of the blood-brain barrier permeability and leakage space using dynamic MR imaging. 1. Fundamental concepts. Magn Reson Med. 1991 Feb;17(2):357-67.

[42] Daldrup HE, Shames DM, Husseini W, Wendland MF, Okuhata Y, Brasch RC. Quantification of the extraction fraction for gadopentetate across breast cancer capillaries. Magn Reson Med. 1998 Oct;40(4):537-43.

[43] Larsson HB, Stubgaard M, Frederiksen JL, Jensen M, Henriksen O, Paulson OB. Quantitation of blood-brain barrier defect by magnetic resonance imaging and gadolinium-DTPA in patients with multiple sclerosis and brain tumors. Magn Reson Med. 1990 Oct;16(1):117-31.

[44] Brix G, Semmler W, Port R, Schad LR, Layer G, Lorenz WJ. Pharmacokinetic parameters in CNS Gd-DTPA enhanced MR imaging. J Comput Assist Tomogr. 1991 Jul-Aug;15(4):621-8.

[45] Boxerman JL, Hamberg LM, Rosen BR, Weisskoff RM. MR contrast due to intravascular magnetic susceptibility perturbations. Magn Reson Med. 1995 Oct;34(4):555-66.

[46] Rosen BR, Belliveau JW, Vevea JM, Brady TJ. Perfusion imaging with NMR contrast agents. Magn Reson Med. 1990 May;14(2):249-65.

[47] Kuppusamy K, Lin W, Cizek GR, Haacke EM. In vivo regional cerebral blood volume: quantitative assessment with 3D T1-weighted pre- and postcontrast MR imaging. Radiology. 1996 Oct;201(1):106-12.

[48] Lin W, Paczynski RP, Kuppusamy K, Hsu CY, Haacke EM. Quantitative measurements of regional cerebral blood volume using MRI in rats: effects of arterial carbon dioxide tension and mannitol. Magn Reson Med. 1997 Sep;38(3):420-8.

[49] Le Duc G, Peoc'h M, Remy C, Charpy O, Muller RN, Le Bas JF, et al. Use of T(2)-weighted susceptibility contrast MRI for mapping the blood volume in the glioma-bearing rat brain. Magn Reson Med. 1999 Oct;42(4):754-61.

[50] Schwarzbauer C, Syha J, Haase A. Quantification of regional blood volumes by rapid T1 mapping. Magn Reson Med. 1993 May;29(5):709-12.

[51] Payen JF, Briot E, Tropres I, Julien-Dolbec C, Montigon O, Decorps M. Regional cerebral blood volume response to hypocapnia using susceptibility contrast MRI. NMR Biomed. 2000 Nov;13(7):384-91.

[52] Tropres I, Lamalle L, Peoc'h M, Farion R, Usson Y, Decorps M, et al. In vivo assessment of tumoral angiogenesis. Magn Reson Med. 2004 Mar;51(3):533-41.

[53] Turetschek K, Floyd E, Helbich T, Roberts TP, Shames DM, Wendland MF, et al. MRI assessment of microvascular characteristics in experimental breast tumors using a new blood pool contrast agent (MS-325) with correlations to histopathology. J Magn Reson Imaging. 2001 Sep;14(3):237-42.

[54] Bereczki D, Wei L, Otsuka T, Acuff V, Pettigrew K, Patlak C, et al. Hypoxia increases velocity of blood flow through parenchymal microvascular systems in rat brain. J Cereb Blood Flow Metab. 1993 May;13(3):475-86.

[55] Cremer JE, Seville MP. Regional brain blood flow, blood volume, and haematocrit values in the adult rat. J Cereb Blood Flow Metab. 1983 Jun;3(2):254-6.

[56] Yablonskiy DA, Haacke EM. Theory of NMR signal behavior in magnetically inhomogeneous tissues: the static dephasing regime. Magn Reson Med. 1994 Dec;32(6):749-63.

[57] Dennie J, Mandeville JB, Boxerman JL, Packard SD, Rosen BR, Weisskoff RM. NMR imaging of changes in vascular morphology due to tumor angiogenesis. Magn Reson Med. 1998 Dec;40(6):793-9.

[58] Lu H, Golay X, Pekar JJ, Van Zijl PC. Functional magnetic resonance imaging based on changes in vascular space occupancy. Magn Reson Med. 2003 Aug;50(2):263-74.

[59] Lu H, Law M, Johnson G, Ge Y, van Zijl PC, Helpern JA. Novel approach to the measurement of absolute cerebral blood volume using vascular-space-occupancy magnetic resonance imaging. Magn Reson Med. 2005 Dec;54(6):1403-11.

[60] Perles-Barbacaru AT, Lahrech H. A new Magnetic Resonance Imaging method for mapping the cerebral blood volume fraction: the rapid steady-state T1 method. J Cereb Blood Flow Metab. 2007 Mar;27(3):618-31.

[61] Haase A. Snapshot FLASH MRI. Applications to T1, T2, and chemical-shift imaging. Magn Reson Med. 1990 Jan;13(1):77-89.

[62] Larsson HB, Stubgaard M, Sondergaard L, Henriksen O. In vivo quantification of the unidirectional influx constant for Gd-DTPA diffusion across the myocardial capillaries with MR imaging. J Magn Reson Imaging. 1994 May-Jun;4(3):433-40.

[63] Jivan A, Horsfield MA, Moody AR, Cherryman GR. Dynamic T1 measurement using snapshot-FLASH MRI. J Magn Reson. 1997 Jul;127(1):65-72.

[64] Fonchy E, Lahrech H, Francois-Joubert A, Dupeyre R, Benderbous S, Corot C, et al. A new gadolinium-based contrast agent for magnetic resonance imaging of brain tumors: kinetic study on a C6 rat glioma model. J Magn Reson Imaging. 2001 Aug; 14(2):97-105.

[65] Perles-Barbacaru AT, Berger F, Lahrech H. Quantitative rapid steady state T(1) magnetic resonance imaging for cerebral blood volume mapping in mice: Lengthened measurement time window with intraperitoneal Gd-DOTA injection. Magn Reson Med 2013 May;69(5);1451-6

[66] Payen JF, Vath A, Koenigsberg B, Bourlier V, Decorps M. Regional cerebral plasma volume response to carbon dioxide using magnetic resonance imaging. Anesthesiology. 1998 Apr;88(4):984-92.

[67] Perles-Barbacaru TA, Procissi D, Demyanenko AV, Jacobs RE. Quantitative pharmacologic MRI in mice. NMR Biomed. 2012 Apr;25(4):498-505.

[68] Shockley RP, LaManna JC. Determination of rat cerebral cortical blood volume changes by capillary mean transit time analysis during hypoxia, hypercapnia and hyperventilation. Brain Res. 1988 Jun 28;454(1-2):170-8.

[69] Beaumont M, Lemasson B, Farion R, Segebarth C, Remy C, Barbier EL. Characterization of tumor angiogenesis in rat brain using iron-based vessel size index MRI in

combination with gadolinium-based dynamic contrast-enhanced MRI. J Cereb Blood Flow Metab. 2009 Oct;29(10):1714-26.

[70] Bremer C, Mustafa M, Bogdanov A, Jr., Ntziachristos V, Petrovsky A, Weissleder R. Steady-state blood volume measurements in experimental tumors with different angiogenic burdens a study in mice. Radiology. 2003 Jan;226(1):214-20.

[71] Julien C, Payen JF, Tropres I, Farion R, Grillon E, Montigon O, et al. Assessment of vascular reactivity in rat brain glioma by measuring regional blood volume during graded hypoxic hypoxia. Br J Cancer. 2004 Jul 19;91(2):374-80.

[72] Valable S, Eddi D, Constans JM, Guillamo JS, Bernaudin M, Roussel S, et al. MRI assessment of hemodynamic effects of angiopoietin-2 overexpression in a brain tumor model. Neuro Oncol. 2009 Oct;11(5):488-502.

[73] Perles-Barbacaru AT, Lamalle L, Barbier E, Segebarth C, Lahrech H, editors. Rapid Steady State T_1 method for cerebral blood volume fraction mapping using SINEREM as contrast agent and a three dimensional projection reconstruction acquisition mode International Society for Magnetic Resonance in Medicine, 16th Annual Scientific Meeting; 2008; Toronto (Canada).

[74] Gadelle A, Defaye J. Selective halogenation of primary positions of cyclomaltosaccharides and synthesis of per-(3,6-anhydro) cyclomalto-oligosacccharides. Angew Chem Int Ed Engl 1991;30(1):78-80.

[75] Lahrech H, Perles-Barbacaru AT, Aous S, Le Bas JF, Debouzy JC, Gadelle A, et al. Cerebral blood volume quantification in a C6 tumor model using gadolinium per (3,6-anhydro) alpha-cyclodextrin as a new magnetic resonance imaging preclinical contrast agent. J Cereb Blood Flow Metab. 2008 May;28(5):1017-29.

[76] Labadie C, Lee JH, Vetek G, Springer CS, Jr. Relaxographic imaging. J Magn Reson B. 1994 Oct;105(2):99-112.

[77] Moran GR, Prato FS. Modeling (1H) exchange: an estimate of the error introduced in MRI by assuming the fast exchange limit in bolus tracking. Magn Reson Med. 2004 Apr;51(4):816-27.

[78] Adair TH, Wells ML, Hang J, Montani JP. A stereological method for estimating length density of the arterial vascular system. Am J Physiol. 1994 Apr;266(4 Pt 2):H1434-8.

[79] Todd MM, Weeks JB, Warner DS. Cerebral blood flow, blood volume, and brain tissue hematocrit during isovolemic hemodilution with hetastarch in rats. Am J Physiol. 1992 Jul;263(1 Pt 2):H75-82.

[80] Todd MM, Weeks JB, Warner DS. The influence of intravascular volume expansion on cerebral blood flow and blood volume in normal rats. Anesthesiology. 1993 May; 78(5):945-53.

[81] Todd MM, Weeks J. Comparative effects of propofol, pentobarbital, and isoflurane on cerebral blood flow and blood volume. J Neurosurg Anesthesiol. 1996 Oct;8(4): 296-303.

[82] Bereczki D, Wei L, Acuff V, Gruber K, Tajima A, Patlak C, et al. Technique-dependent variations in cerebral microvessel blood volumes and hematocrits in the rat. J Appl Physiol. 1992 Sep;73(3):918-24.

[83] Lin W, Celik A, Paczynski RP, Hsu CY, Powers WJ. Quantitative magnetic resonance imaging in experimental hypercapnia: improvement in the relation between changes in brain R2 and the oxygen saturation of venous blood after correction for changes in cerebral blood volume. J Cereb Blood Flow Metab. 1999 Aug;19(8):853-62.

[84] Dunn JF, Roche MA, Springett R, Abajian M, Merlis J, Daghlian CP, et al. Monitoring angiogenesis in brain using steady-state quantification of DeltaR2 with MION infusion. Magn Reson Med. 2004 Jan;51(1):55-61.

[85] Schwarzbauer C, Morrissey SP, Deichmann R, Hillenbrand C, Syha J, Adolf H, et al. Quantitative magnetic resonance imaging of capillary water permeability and regional blood volume with an intravascular MR contrast agent. Magn Reson Med. 1997 May;37(5):769-77.

[86] Julien-Dolbec C, Tropres I, Montigon O, Reutenauer H, Ziegler A, Decorps M, et al. Regional response of cerebral blood volume to graded hypoxic hypoxia in rat brain. Br J Anaesth. 2002 Aug;89(2):287-93.

[87] Tropres I, Grimault S, Vaeth A, Grillon E, Julien C, Payen JF, et al. Vessel size imaging. Magn Reson Med. 2001 Mar;45(3):397-408.

[88] Pathak AP, Schmainda KM, Ward BD, Linderman JR, Rebro KJ, Greene AS. MR-derived cerebral blood volume maps: issues regarding histological validation and assessment of tumor angiogenesis. Magn Reson Med. 2001 Oct;46(4):735-47.

[89] Adam JF, Elleaume H, Le Duc G, Corde S, Charvet AM, Tropres I, et al. Absolute cerebral blood volume and blood flow measurements based on synchrotron radiation quantitative computed tomography. J Cereb Blood Flow Metab. 2003 Apr;23(4): 499-512.

[90] Verant P, Serduc R, Van Der Sanden B, Remy C, Vial JC. A direct method for measuring mouse capillary cortical blood volume using multiphoton laser scanning microscopy. J Cereb Blood Flow Metab. 2007 May;27(5):1072-81.

Chapter 8

FDG- PET Imaging in Neurodegenerative Brain Diseases

L. K. Teune, A. L. Bartels and K. L. Leenders

Additional information is available at the end of the chapter

1. Introduction

1.1. Cerebral glucose metabolism

Increases and decreases of synaptic activity in the brain are accompanied by proportional changes in capillary perfusion and local glucose consumption. These changes in glucose consumption are the effect of changed activity or density of the afferent nerve terminals in that region. Loss of neurons may result in decreased glucose consumption in distant brain regions by deafferentiation, while also increased regional glucose consumption by increased activation of afferent neurons can occur. The PET tracer [18F]fluorodeoxyglucose (FDG) allows the measurement of glucose consumption. FDG is a glucose analog with physiological aspects almost identical to glucose. It is transported from the blood to the brain by a carrier-mediated diffusion mechanism. FDG and glucose are phosphorylated by hexokinase as the first step of the glycolytic process. FDG differs from glucose in that a hydrogen atom replaced the hydroxyl group at the second carbon atom of the molecule. Glucose is then phosphorylated to glucose-6-PO_4, and continues along the glycolytic pathway for energy production. However, FDG is phosphorylated to FDG-6-PO_4, which is not a substrate for further metabolism and trapped in tissues. As glucose is the only source of energy for the brain it reflects the neuronal integrity of underlying brain pathology. Since FDG is a competitive substrate with glucose for both transport and phosphorylation, it is important for tracer uptake to avoid high blood glucose levels during an FDG-PET scan in subjects with diabetes.

In neurodegenerative brain diseases, specific brain regions degenerate and specific patterns of metabolic brain activity develop. This happens before clear structural changes can be detected with imaging techniques.

Measurement of glucose consumption with FDG PET imaging thus allows us to identify disease-specific cerebral metabolic brain patterns in several neurodegenerative brain diseases at an early disease stage. Since the first FDG PET study in man in 1979 (Reivich, et al. 1979)

regional differences in cerebral glucose metabolism have been reported in various neurodegenerative brain diseases including parkinsonian syndromes.

2. Disease-specific metabolic brain patterns: Methods

Univariate methods like voxel-based statistical parametric mapping (SPM) analyses have been used to identify group differences between patients with neurodegenerative brain diseases and controls. (Eckert, et al. 2005, Juh, et al. 2004, Yong, et al. 2007).

At the University Medical Center Groningen, The Netherlands we have performed a retrospective study (Teune, et al. 2010) selecting typical patients with 7 different neurodegenerative brain diseases who had had a clinical FDG brain scan at a time point when their diagnosis was not sure yet. These patients developed in the following years the mentioned typical disease states. Images of each of the seven patient groups were separately compared to controls using a two-sample t test. At those early scans, already typical differences between patient - and control groups were found for each disease.

However, Scaled Subprofile modelling/principal component analysis (SSM/PCA), a multivariate method, not only identifies group differences, but is also able to identify relationships in relatively increased and decreased metabolic activity between different brain regions in combined samples of patients and control scans (Eidelberg. 2009, Moeller, et al. 1987). Covariance analysis techniques are considered appropriate methods to explore network activity. In the SSM, a threshold of the whole-brain maximum can be applied to remove out-of-brain voxels, followed by a log transformation. A threshold of 35% is used by the Eidelberg research group resulting in a mask of mainly grey matter (Spetsieris and Eidelberg. 2010). After removing between-subject and between-region averages, a principal component analysis (PCA) can be applied. PCA transformes a set of correlated variables into a new set of orthogonal uncorrelated variables that are called the principal components. Voxels participating in each principal component (PC) may have either a positive or a negative loading. The loadings express the covariance structure (i.e. the strength of the interaction) between the voxels that participate in the PC. They are ordered in terms of the variability they represent. That is, the first principal components represents for a single dimension (variable) the greatest amount of variability in the original dataset. Each succeeding orthogonal component accounts for as much of the remaining variability as possible. They can be very helpful in determining how many of the components are really significant and how much the data can be reduced.

In most studies, the components that together describe at least 50% of the variance are used for further analysis, but this is an arbitrary limit. To identify a covariance pattern that best discriminates a patient group from a control group, each subject's expression of the selected principal components with the lowest AIC (Akaike information criterion) value (Akaike. 1974) are entered into a stepwise regression procedure. This regression results in a linear combination of the PCs that best discriminated the two groups and is designated as the disease-specific metabolic covariance pattern.

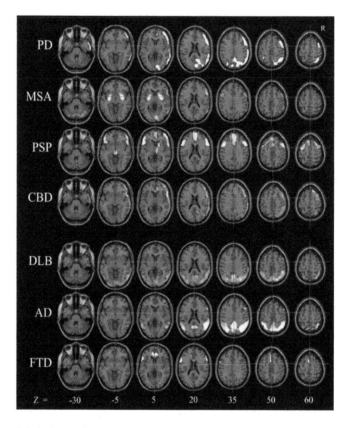

Figure 1. Typical cerebral metabolic patterns in neurodegenerative brain diseases. SPM (t) maps of decreased metabolic activity were overlaid on a T1 MR template thresholded at P< 0.001 with cluster cutoff of 20 voxels. Patient groups are indicated on the vertical axis and on the horizontal axis, seven transversal slices through the brain are shown. PD = Parkinson's disease: decreased metabolic activity in the contralateral to the most affected body side parieto-occipital and frontal regions; MSA = multiple system atrophy: decreased metabolic activity in bilateral putamen and cerebellum; PSP = progressive supranuclear palsy: decreased metabolic activity in the prefrontal cortex, caudate nucleus, thalamus and mesencephalon; CBD = corticobasal degeneration: decreased metabolic activity in the contralateral to the most affected body side cortical regions; DLB = dementia with Lewy bodies: decreased metabolic activity in the occipital and parieto-temporal regions. AD = Alzheimer's Disease: decreased metabolic activity in the angular gyrus and other parieto-temporal regions including precuneus extending to the posterior- and middle cingulate gyrus. FTD = frontotemporal dementia: decreased metabolic activity in the superior and inferior frontal gyrus, anterior cingulate gyrus, SMA, sensorimotor area and middle temporal gyrus. Adapted from: Teune et al. (2010) Typical cerebral metabolic patterns in neurodegenerative brain diseases. Movement Disorders. 2010;25:2395-404.

Important for its use in clinical practice is that this metabolic covariance pattern can then be applied to individual patients to test whether they express the pattern or not. Every voxel value in a subject scan is multiplied by the corresponding voxel weight in the covariance pattern, with a subsequent summation over the whole brain volume. The resulting subject score captures to what extent a subject expresses the covariance pattern.

3. Disease-specific metabolic brain patterns in patients with parkinsonism

3.1. Parkinson's disease

Parkinson's disease (PD) is characterized by bradykinesia, rigidity, sometimes rest tremor and postural instability. A disturbed α-synuclein protein forming so-called Lewy bodies seems to play a causal role, which was a reason to designate PD as a α-synucleinopathy. The main pathophysiological changes result from degeneration of catecholaminergic, especially dopaminergic cells in brainstem regions.

A characteristic metabolic covariance pattern has been identified in PD patients (PD-related pattern, PDRP) showing regionally relatively increased metabolism in the globus pallidus and putamen, thalamus, pons and cerebellum and relatively decreased metabolism in the lateral frontal, premotor and parietal association areas (Ma, et al. 2007) Network expression in PD patients also increases linearly with disease progression(Huang, et al. 2007b). Tang et al. tried to study network changes in the PD-related motor pattern before symptom onset by studying 15 hemiparkinsonian patients and focusing mainly on the "presymptomatic" hemisphere. They conclude that abnormal PDRP activity antecedes the appearance of motor signs by approximately 2 years (Tang, et al. 2010a). However, this needs to be proven in future research in true presymptomatic patients.

3.2. Parkinson's disease and metabolic brain patterns related to specific symptoms

In addition to motor symptoms, cognitive dysfunction is also common in PD, especially executive and visuospatial dysfunction. FDG-PET studies have been performed to study these specific symptoms and their relations with neural network pathophysiology. The Eidelberg research group has shown PD subclassifications related to specific symptoms. Network analysis with the SSM/PCA approach detected a significant covariance pattern in non-demented PD patients that correlated with memory and executive functioning tasks. The expression of this PD-related cognitive pattern (PDCP) in individual patients correlated with severity of cognitive dysfunction(Huang, et al. 2007a).

Alterations in neuropsychological test results in advanced PD were found to correlate with decreases in glucose metabolism in the dorsolateral prefrontal cortex (DLPFC), lateral orbitofrontal cortex (LOFC) ventral and dorsal cingulum (v/dACC) and in Broca area (Kalbe, et al. 2009). In the study of Kalbe et al, PD patients with deep brain stimulation in the subthalamic nucleus (STN-DBS) showed cognitive decline that correlated with decrease in glucose metabolism in these areas. In another study in STN-DBS treated patients, STN DBS was found to activate glucose metabolism in the frontal limbic and associative territory (Hilker, et al. 2004). Interestingly, cortical areas that show hypometabolism in patients with depression (Mayberg HS. 1994) are similar to the regions that show restored glucose metabolism after STN DBS. This finding agrees with the clinical observation that PD-related depression tends to improve after STN DBS.

Mure et al. identified a spatial covariance pattern associated with Parkinson tremor which was characterized by covarying increases in the cerebellum/dentate nucleus and primary cortex and to a minor degree in the caudate/putamen (Mure, et al. 2011).

Hallucinations in PD have been related to relative frontal hypermetabolism compared to PD patients without hallucinations(Nagano-Saito, et al. 2004). However, another study showed hypometabolism in occipitotemporoparietal regions in PD patients with hallucinations, sparing the occipital pole, while no significant increase in regional glucose metabolism was detected (Boecker, et al. 2007). Interestingly, in patients with dementia with Lewy bodies (DLB), who also suffer from hallucinations, glucose metabolism was also decreased in occipitoparietal regions, however without sparing of the occipital pole (see DLB section).

3.3. Multiple system atrophy

Multiple system atrophy is a sporadic neurodegenerative brain disease which affects both men and women and generally starts in the sixth decade of life. The main clinical features are parkinsonism, autonomic failure, cerebellar ataxia, and pyramidal signs in any combination. However, two major motor presentations can be distinguished. Parkinsonian features predominate in 80% of patients (MSA-P subtype) and cerebellar ataxia is the main motor feature in 20% of patients (MSA-C subtype) ((Gilman, et al. 2008, Wenning, et al. 1997)

In MSA-P the striatonigral system is the main site of pathology but less severe degeneration can be widespread and normally includes the olivopontocerebellar system. In MSA-C pathological changes are mainly seen in the olivopontocerebellar system and involvement of striatum and substantia nigra are less severe (Wenning, et al. 1997). The discovery of glial cytoplasmic inclusions in MSA brains highlighted the unique glial pathology as biological hallmark of the disease. Their distribution selectively involves basal ganglia, supplementary and primary motor cortex, the reticular formation and pontocerebellar system. Glial cytoplasmic inclusions contain besides classical cytoskeletal antigens also α-synuclein, which is a presynaptic protein present in Lewy Bodies, and this accumulation seems to play a central part not only in MSA but also in other α-synucleinopathies such as PD and DLB.

Disease-related metabolic patterns were also present in MSA consisting of hypometabolism in putamen and cerebellum in MSA (Eckert, et al. 2008). Poston et al. found that differences in expression of the MSA-related pattern correlated with clinical disability (Poston, et al. 2012).

3.4. Progressive supranuclear palsy

The clinical picture of progressive supranuclear palsy (PSP) has been first described by Steele, Richardson and Olszewski (Steele JC, Richardson J,Olszewski J. 1964) and is characterized by progressive parkinsonism, early gait and balance impairment, vertical gaze palsy and more profound frontal cognitive disturbances. PSP is one of several neurodegenerative diseases characterised by accumulation of hyperphosphorylated tau (tauopathy), forming abnormal filamentous inclusions in neurons and glia in the precentral and postcentral cortical areas but also in the thalamus, subthalamic nucleus, red nucleus and substantia nigra. Other neurodegenerative brain diseases which show disturbances in tau protein handling are corticobasal degeneration (CBD) and frontotemporal dementia (FTD) but there is also overlap in pathology with Alzheimer's disease (AD).

However the metabolic brain patterns in these tauopathies are quite different. The covariance pattern of PSP consists of decreased metabolism in the prefrontal cortex, frontal eye fields, caudate nuclei, medial thalamus and upper brainstem (Eckert, et al. 2008). Brain stem atrophy and atrophy of the medial frontal cortical regions have also been reported in histopathological studies (Hauw, et al. 1994).

3.5. Corticobasal degeneration

The most striking features of patients with corticobasal degeneration (CBD) include marked asymmetrical parkinsonism and apraxia but also postural instability, limb dystonia, cortical sensory loss, dementia and the alien limb phenomenon. CBD is one of the tauopathies and clinical diagnosis is complicated by both the variability of presentation of true CBD and the syndromes that look alike but are caused by other tauopathies with parkinsonism like PSP or FTD (Josephs, et al. 2006). However with functional neuroimaging a clear distinction can be made. In CBD a typical pattern of hypometabolism is seen in cortical regions contralateral to the affected body side, including parieto-temporal regions, prefrontal cortex and motor cortex. Furthermore, a decrease can be found in the contralateral caudate nucleus, putamen and thalamus (Eckert, et al. 2005, Teune, et al. 2010). No covariance pattern has been described using the SSM/PCA technique in CBD.

4. Disease-specific metabolic brain patterns in the differential diagnosis of individual patients with parkinsonism

Interestingly, Tang and co-workers studied the potential role of FDG PET in the individual diagnosis of 167 patients who had parkinsonian features but uncertain clinical diagnosis (Tang, et al. 2010b) After FDG PET imaging, patients were assessed by blinded movement disorders specialists for a mean of 2.6 years before a final clinical diagnosis was made (gold standard). SSM/PCA analysis can quantify the expression of an obtained covariance pattern in each subject which allows assessing the expression of a given pattern on a single case basis. Using this automated image-based classification procedure and the previously defined disease related covariance patterns in PD, MSA and PSP, individual patients were differentiated with high specificity.

However, blinded, prospective imaging studies (ideally involving multiple centers, a larger validation group, repeat imaging, and more extensive post-mortem confirmation) are needed to establish the accuracy and precision of this pattern-based categorisation procedure. These studies are currently undertaken.

For routine clinical practice, this knowledge of disease specific patterns of regional metabolic activity in neurodegenerative brain diseases can be a valuable aid in the differential diagnosis of individual patients, especially at an early disease stage.

5. Disease-specific metabolic brain patterns in dementia

5.1. Alzheimer's disease

Alzheimer's disease (AD) is a progressive neurodegenerative brain disease accounting for 50-60% of cases of dementia. AD is characterized by a severe decline in episodic memory together with general cognitive symptoms such as impaired judgement, decision making and orientation (McKhann, et al. 1984). A correct clinical diagnosis can be difficult, especially in early disease stages or in patients with for example comorbid depression, high education or young age (Bohnen, et al. 2012). FDG-PET imaging can be used to assist in the differential diagnosis, because for different dementia syndromes, a separate pattern of hypometabolism can be found. In Alzheimer's disease (AD), decline of FDG uptake in posterior cingulate, temporoparietal and prefrontal association cortex was related to dementia severity (Herholz, et al. 2002). Foster et al used visual interpretation of an automated three-dimensional stereo-tactic surface projection technique of patients with AD and FTD. They showed that visual interpretation of FDG-PET scans after training is more reliable and accurate in distinguishing FTD from AD than clinical methods alone (Foster, et al. 2007).

Although multivariate analytical techniques might identify diagnostic patterns that are not captured by univariate methods, they have rarely been used to study neural correlates of Alzheimer's Disease or cognitive impairment. Because cognitive processes are the result of integrated activity in networks rather than activity of any one area in isolation, functional connectivity can be better captured by multivariate methods. A study from Habeck et al. examined the efficacy of multivariate and univariate analytical methods and concluded that multivariate analysis might be more sensitive than univariate analysis for the diagnosis of early Alzheimer's disease (Habeck, et al. 2008).

Scarmeas et al. were the first to derive an AD related covariance pattern using $H_2^{15}O$ to measure brain perfusion (Scarmeas, et al. 2004). It consisted of relatively increased perfusion in the bilateral insula, lingual gyri and cuneus with bilaterally decreased flow in bilateral inferior parietal lobule and cingulate in AD patients. However, using this PET tracer they found a sensitivity of 76-94% and a specificity of 63-81% with considerable overlap in pattern expression among AD patients and controls. Therefore they concluded that the derived $H_2^{15}O$ pattern cannot be used as a sufficient diagnostic test in clinical settings. Specific FDG covariance patterns to distinguish early AD-related cognitive decline using multivariate methods have yet to be specified.

5.2. Frontotemporal dementia

Frontotemporal dementia (FTD) is one of the neurodegenerative diseases commonly mistaken for AD. FTD patients do not have a true amnestic syndrome but can present with either gradual and progressive changes in behaviour, or gradual and progressive language dysfunction. Gross examination of the post-mortem brain from a patient with FTD usually reveals frontal or temporal lobar atrophy or both, but the distribution or severity of brain atrophy are not specific for a particular neurodegenerative brain disease. Jeong et al. and Diehl-Schmid et al.

analysed FDG-PET scans of FTD patients on a voxel-by-voxel basis using Statistical Parametric Mapping (SPM). They found hypometabolism depending on disease stage in the frontal lobe, parietal and temporal cortices (Diehl-Schmid, et al. 2007, Jeong, et al. 2005).

5.3. Dementia with Lewy Bodies

The clinical overlap of dementia and parkinsonism is highlighted in Dementia with Lewy Bodies (DLB). These patients show besides dementia extrapyramidal motor symptoms and marked neuropsychiatric disturbances including visual hallucinations, depression, variability in arousal and attention (McKeith. 2006). Consistent observation of a metabolic reduction in the medial occipital cortex in DLB patients (Minoshima, et al. 2001, Teune, et al. 2010) using FDG-PET imaging suggests the use of FDG-PET in the differential diagnosis of AD and DLB and of PD and DLB. Minoshima et al. found that the presence of occipital hypometabolism distinguished DLB from AD with 90% sensitivity and 80% specificity when using post-mortem diagnosis as the gold standard diagnosis (Minoshima, et al. 2001).

6. Disease-specific metabolic brain patterns in hyperkinetic movement disorders

6.1. Huntington's disease

Huntington's disease (HD) is characterized by progressive dementia and chorea, starting around 30-40 years of age. HD is caused by a dominantly inherited CAG repeat expansion mutation that generates lengthening of the protein huntingtin, with size-dependent neuro-toxicity. Several PET studies have shown hypometabolism in the caudate nucleus, both in symptomatic and asymptomatic mutation carriers (Grafton, et al. 1992) (Antonini A., et al. 1996) In asymptomatic carriers, metabolic decreases were also significantly associated with the CAG repeat number (Antonini A., et al. 1996). Furthermore, it was found that FDG uptake in the caudate nucleus provided a predictive measure for time of onset of the disease, in addition to the mutation size (Ciarmiello A., et al. 2012).

Another study applied network analysis of FDG-PET scans in presymptomatic mutation carriers (Feigin, et al. 2001). They found a HD related metabolic covariance pattern (HDRP) characterized by caudate and putamenal hypometabolism, but also including mediotemporal reductions as well as relative increases in occipital regions. Disturbances of these striatotemporal projections may underlie aspects of the psychiatric and cognitive abnormalities that occur in the earliest stages of HD, before the onset of motor signs (Cummings JL. 1995).

6.2. Dystonia

Dystonia is a movement disorder characterized by involuntary, sustained muscle contractions causing twisting movements and abnormal postures. The most common forms of primary torsion dystonia (PTD) are DYT1 and DYT6, both caused by autosomal inherited mutations with a reduced penetrance.

Functional neuroimaging techniques have been applied in different dystonic disorders including primary generalized dystonia, mainly DYT1 and DYT6 and dopa-responsive dystonia, as well as focal dystonic syndromes such as torticollis, writer's cramp and blepharospasm. A common finding is abnormality of the basal ganglia, cerebellum and associated outflow pathways to sensorimotor cortex and other regions involved with motor performance. However, controversial results have been found in imaging dystonias, partly attributed to methodological differences but also to the heterogeneity of the dystonias. Using the SSM/PCA approach a reproducible pattern of abnormal regional glucose utilization in two independent cohorts of DYT1 carriers have been found (Eidelberg D. 1998)(Trost M., et al. 2002).

This torsion-dystonia related metabolic pattern is characterized by increases in the posterior putamen/globus pallidus, cerebellum and SMA. Interestingly, also in clinically non-manifesting mutation carriers this pattern was found, suggesting a cerebral "vulnerability to develop dystonia" network change. Also in manifesting and non-manifesting DYT 6 carriers abnormal network activity has been identified. A difference between DYT1 and DYT6 metabolic patterns can be seen in the putamen, where glucose metabolism is increased in DYT1 and decreased in DYT6, possibly do to cell loss in DYT6. Furthermore, the cerebellum shows increased activity in DYT1 and normal activity in DYT6 (Carbon M., et al. 2004).

The TDRP network is not expressed in patients with Dopa-responsive dystonia (DRD) (Trost M., et al. 2002).

DRD is characterized by an early onset of dystonic symptoms and later appearance of parkinsonian symptoms. A defining feature is a marked and sustained response to low doses of levodopa, suggesting that the lesion may be functional in the presynaptic dopaminergic system rather than anatomical. The DRD related metabolic pattern is characterized by relative increases in the dorsal midbrain, cerebellar vermis,and SMA, assiocated with covarying decreases in putamen, lateral premotor and motor cortical regions (Asanuma, et al. 2005b). This DRD related pattern is not apparent in DYT 1 and 6 carriers supporting the hypothesis that the pathophysiology of DRD differs from that of other forms of dystonia. They also found that the Parkinson-related metabolic pattern is not apparent in DRD patients. Thus FDG-PET can be useful to distinguish PD related dystonia from dopa-responsive dystonia with parkinsonism (Asanuma, et al. 2005a).

6.3. Gilles de la Tourette

Tourette syndrome is characterized by the presence of chronic motor and vocal tics that develop before the age of 18. Comorbid behavioural abnormalities are common in Tourette syndrome, most notably obsessive-compulsive disorder and attention deficit/hyperactivity disorder (Lebowitz, et al. 2012). The neurophysiology remains poorly understood with varying and inconsistent neuropathological and neuroimaging findings, possibly due to the clinical heterogeneity of the disorder. Pourfar et al. identified a Tourette syndrome related pattern characterized by reduced metabolic activity of the striatum and orbitofrontal cortex associated with relatively increased metabolic activity in the premotor cortex and cerebellum. A second metabolic brain pattern was found in patients with Tourette syndrome and obsessive compulsive disorder characterized by reduced activity in the anterior cingulate and dorsolateral prefrontal cortex and relative increases in primary motor cortex and precuneus. Subject expression correlated with symptom severity. These findings suggest that the different clinical manifestations of the Tourette syndrome are associated with different abnormal brain networks (Pourfar, et al. 2011).

7. Conclusion

FDG-PET imaging is increasingly available for routine clinical practice and has remained the only available radiotracer to detect accurately and reliably the cerebral glucose metabolism. As glucose is the only source of energy for the brain it reflects the energy needs of underlying brain neuronal systems. The SSM/PCA method can identify relationships in relatively increased and decreased metabolic activity between different brain regions in combined samples of patients and controls. The expression of an obtained covariance pattern can be quantified in an individual patient and this resulting subject score captures to what extent a patient expresses the covariance patterns. The disease-related metabolic brain patterns can therefore be a valuable aid in the early differential diagnosis of individual patients with neurodegenerative brain diseases.

Author details

L. K. Teune, A. L. Bartels* and K. L. Leenders

*Address all correspondence to: a.l.bartels@umcg.nl

Department of Neurology, University Medical Center Groningen, The Netherlands

References

[1] Akaike, H. A new look at the statistical model identification. A New Look at the Statistical Model Identification (1974). , 1974, 716-23.

[2] Antonini, A, Leenders, K. L, Spiegel, R, Meier, D, Vontobel, P, Weigell-weber, M, et al. Striatal glucose metabolism and dopamine D2 receptor binding in asymptomatic gene carriers and patients with huntington's disease. (1996).

[3] Asanuma, K, Carbon-correll, M, & Eidelberg, D. Neuroimaging in human dystonia. (2005a).

[4] Asanuma, K, Ma, Y, Huang, C, Carbon-correll, M, Edwards, C, Raymond, D, et al. The metabolic pathology of dopa-responsive dystonia. (2005b).

[5] Boecker, H, Ceballos-baumann, A. O, Volk, D, Conrad, B, Forstl, H, & Haussermann, P. Metabolic alterations in patients with parkinson disease and visual hallucinations. Arch Neurol (2007). , 64, 984-8.

[6] Bohnen, N. I. Djang DSW, Herholz K, Anzai Y, Minoshima S. Effectiveness and safety of 18F-FDG PET in the evaluation of dementia: A review of the recent literature. Journal of Nuclear Medicine (2012). , 53, 59-71.

[7] Carbon, M, Trost, M, Ghilardi, M. F, & Eidelberg, D. Abnormal brain networks in primary torsion dystonia. (2004).

[8] Ciarmiello, A, Giovacchini, G, Orobello, S, Bruselli, L, Elifani, F, & Squitieri, F. F-FDG PET uptake in the pre-huntington disease caudate affects the time-to-onset independently of CAG expansion size. (2012).

[9] Cummings, J. L. Behavioral and psychiatric symptoms associated with huntington's disease. (1995).

[10] Diehl-schmid, J, Grimmer, T, Drzezga, A, Bornschein, S, Riemenschneider, M, Forstl, H, et al. Decline of cerebral glucose metabolism in frontotemporal dementia: A longitudinal 18F-FDG-PET-study. Neurobiol Aging (2007). , 28, 42-50.

[11] Eckert, T, Barnes, A, Dhawan, V, Frucht, S, Gordon, M. F, Feigin, A. S, et al. FDG PET in the differential diagnosis of parkinsonian disorders. Neuroimage (2005). , 26, 912-21.

[12] Eckert, T, Tang, C, Ma, Y, Brown, N, Lin, T, Frucht, S, et al. Abnormal metabolic networks in atypical parkinsonism. Mov Disord (2008).

[13] Eidelberg, D. Abnormal brain networks in DYT1 dystonia. (1998).

[14] Eidelberg, D. Metabolic brain networks in neurodegenerative disorders: A functional imaging approach. Trends Neurosci (2009). , 32, 548-57.

[15] Feigin, A, Leenders, K. L, Moeller, J. R, Missimer, J, Kuenig, G, Spetsieris, P, et al. Metabolic network abnormalities in early huntington's disease: An [(18)F]FDG PET study. J Nucl Med (2001). , 42, 1591-5.

[16] Foster, N. L, Heidebrink, J. L, Clark, C. M, Jagust, W. J, Arnold, S. E, Barbas, N. R, et al. FDG-PET improves accuracy in distinguishing frontotemporal dementia and alzheimer's disease. Brain (2007). , 130, 2616-35.

[17] Gilman, S, Wenning, G. K, Low, P. A, Brooks, D. J, Mathias, C. J, Trojanowski, J. Q, et al. Second consensus statement on the diagnosis of multiple system atrophy. Neurology (2008). , 71, 670-6.

[18] Grafton, S. T, Mazziotta, J. C, & Pahl, J. J. St George-Hyslop P, Haines JL, Gusella J, et al. Serial changes of cerebral glucose metabolism and caudate size in persons at risk for huntington's disease. (1992).

[19] Habeck, C, Foster, N. L, Perneczky, R, Kurz, A, Alexopoulos, P, Koeppe, R. A, et al. Multivariate and univariate neuroimaging biomarkers of alzheimer's disease. Neuro-image (2008). , 40, 1503-15.

[20] Hauw, J. J, Daniel, S. E, Dickson, D, Horoupian, D. S, Jellinger, K, Lantos, P. L, et al. Preliminary NINDS neuropathologic criteria for steele-richardson-olszewski syndrome (progressive supranuclear palsy). Neurology (1994). , 44, 2015-9.

[21] Herholz, K, Salmon, E, Perani, D, Baron, J. C, Holthoff, V, Frolich, L, et al. Discrimination between alzheimer dementia and controls by automated analysis of multicenter FDG PET. Neuroimage (2002). , 17, 302-16.

[22] Hilker, R, Voges, J, Weisenbach, S, Kalbe, E, Burghaus, L, Ghaemi, M, et al. Subthalamic nucleus stimulation restores glucose metabolism in associative and limbic cortices and in cerebellum: Evidence from a FDG-PET study in advanced parkinson's disease. J Cereb Blood Flow Metab (2004). , 24, 7-16.

[23] Huang, C, Eidelberg, D, Habeck, C, Moeller, J, Svensson, L, Tarabula, T, et al. Imaging markers of mild cognitive impairment: Multivariate analysis of CBF SPECT. Neurobiol Aging (2007a). , 28, 1062-9.

[24] Huang, C, Tang, C, Feigin, A, Lesser, M, Ma, Y, Pourfar, M, et al. Changes in network activity with the progression of parkinson's disease. Brain (2007b). , 130, 1834-46.

[25] Jeong, Y, Cho, S. S, Park, J. M, Kang, S. J, Lee, J. S, Kang, E, et al. F-FDG PET findings in frontotemporal dementia: An SPM analysis of 29 patients. J Nucl Med (2005). , 46, 233-9.

[26] Josephs, K. A, Petersen, R. C, Knopman, D. S, Boeve, B. F, Whitwell, J. L, Duffy, J. R, et al. Clinicopathologic analysis of frontotemporal and corticobasal degenerations and PSP. Neurology (2006). , 66, 41-8.

[27] Juh, R, Kim, J, Moon, D, Choe, B, & Suh, T. Different metabolic patterns analysis of parkinsonism on the 18F-FDG PET. Eur J Radiol (2004). , 51, 223-33.

[28] Kalbe, E, Voges, J, Weber, T, Haarer, M, Baudrexel, S, Klein, J. C, et al. Frontal FDG-PET activity correlates with cognitive outcome after STN-DBS in parkinson disease. Neurology (2009). , 72, 42-9.

[29] Lebowitz, E. R, Motlagh, M. G, Katsovich, L, King, R. A, Lombroso, P. J, Grantz, H, et al. Tourette syndrome in youth with and without obsessive compulsive disorder and attention deficit hyperactivity disorder. (2012).

[30] Ma, Y, Tang, C, Spetsieris, P. G, Dhawan, V, & Eidelberg, D. Abnormal metabolic network activity in parkinson's disease: Test-retest reproducibility. Journal of cerebral blood flow and metabolism : official journal of the International Society of Cerebral Blood Flow and Metabolism (2007). , 27, 597-605.

[31] Mayberg, H. S. Frontal lobe dysfunction in secondary depression. (1994).

[32] Mckeith, I. G. Consensus guidelines for the clinical and pathologic diagnosis of de-
      mentia with lewy bodies (DLB): Report of the consortium on DLB international
      workshop. J Alzheimers Dis (2006). , 9, 417-23.

[33] Mckhann, G, Drachman, D, Folstein, M, Katzman, R, Price, D, & Stadlan, E. M. Clini-
      cal diagnosis of alzheimer's disease: Report of the NINCDS-ADRDA work group un-
      der the auspices of department of health and human services task force on
      alzheimer's disease 35. Neurology (1984). , 34, 939-44.

[34] Minoshima, S, Foster, N. L, Sima, A. A, Frey, K. A, Albin, R. L, & Kuhl, D. E. Alz-
      heimer's disease versus dementia with lewy bodies: Cerebral metabolic distinction
      with autopsy confirmation. Ann Neurol (2001). , 50, 358-65.

[35] Moeller, J. R, Strother, S. C, Sidtis, J. J, & Rottenberg, D. A. Scaled subprofile model:
      A statistical approach to the analysis of functional patterns in positron emission to-
      mographic data. J Cereb Blood Flow Metab (1987). , 7, 649-58.

[36] Mure, H, Hirano, S, Tang, C. C, Isaias, I. U, Antonini, A, Ma, Y, et al. Parkinson's dis-
      ease tremor-related metabolic network: Characterization, progression, and treatment
      effects. Neuroimage (2011). , 54, 1244-53.

[37] Nagano-saito, A, Washimi, Y, Arahata, Y, Iwai, K, Kawatsu, S, Ito, K, et al. Visual
      hallucination in parkinson's disease with FDG PET. Mov Disord (2004). , 19, 801-6.

[38] Poston, K. L, Tang, C. C, Eckert, T, Dhawan, V, Frucht, S, Vonsattel, J, et al. Network
      correlates of disease severity in multiple system atrophy. Neurology (2012). , 78,
      1237-44.

[39] Pourfar, M, Feigin, A, Tang, C. C, Carbon-correll, M, Bussa, M, Budman, C, et al. Ab-
      normal metabolic brain networks in tourette syndrome. Neurology (2011). , 76,
      944-52.

[40] Reivich, M, Kuhl, D, Wolf, A, Greenberg, J, Phelps, M, Ido, T, et al. The [18F]fluoro-
      deoxyglucose method for the measurement of local cerebral glucose utilization in
      man. Circ Res (1979). , 44, 127-37.

[41] Scarmeas, N, Habeck, C. G, Zarahn, E, Anderson, K. E, Park, A, Hilton, J, et al. Cova-
      riance PET patterns in early alzheimer's disease and subjects with cognitive impair-
      ment but no dementia: Utility in group discrimination and correlations with
      functional performance. Neuroimage (2004). , 23, 35-45.

[42] Spetsieris, P. G, & Eidelberg, D. Scaled subprofile modeling of resting state imaging
      data in parkinson's disease: Methodological issues. Neuroimage (2010).

[43] Steele, J. C, Richardson, J, & Olszewski, J. Progressive supranuclear palsy: A hetero-
      geneous degeneration involving the brain stem, basal ganglia and cerebellum with
      vertical gaze and pseudobulbar palsy, nuchal dystonia and dementia. Archives of
      Neurology (1964). , 10, 333-59.

[44] Tang, C. C, Poston, K. L, Dhawan, V, & Eidelberg, D. Abnormalities in metabolic network activity precede the onset of motor symptoms in parkinson's disease. J Neurosci (2010a). , 30, 1049-56.

[45] Tang, C. C, Poston, K. L, Eckert, T, Feigin, A, Frucht, S, Gudesblatt, M, et al. Differential diagnosis of parkinsonism: A metabolic imaging study using pattern analysis. Lancet Neurol (2010b). , 9, 149-58.

[46] Teune, L. K, Bartels, A. L, De Jong, B. M, Willemsen, A. T, Eshuis, S. A, De Vries, J. J, et al. Typical cerebral metabolic patterns in neurodegenerative brain diseases. Mov Disord (2010). , 25, 2395-404.

[47] Trost, M, Carbon, M, Edwards, C, Ma, Y, Raymond, D, Mentis, M. J, et al. Primary dystonia: Is abnormal functional brain architecture linked to genotype? (2002).

[48] Wenning, G. K, & Tison, F. Ben Shlomo Y, Daniel SE, Quinn NP. Multiple system atrophy: A review of 203 pathologically proven cases. Mov Disord (1997). , 12, 133-47.

[49] Yong, S. W, Yoon, J. K, An, Y. S, & Lee, P. H. A comparison of cerebral glucose metabolism in parkinson's disease, parkinson's disease dementia and dementia with lewy bodies. Eur J Neurol (2007). , 14, 1357-62.

Permissions

The contributors of this book come from diverse backgrounds, making this book a truly international effort. This book will bring forth new frontiers with its revolutionizing research information and detailed analysis of the nascent developments around the world.

We would like to thank Prof. Francesco Signorelli and Prof. Domenico Chirchiglia, for lending their expertise to make the book truly unique. They have played a crucial role in the development of this book. Without their invaluable contribution this book wouldn't have been possible. They have made vital efforts to compile up to date information on the varied aspects of this subject to make this book a valuable addition to the collection of many professionals and students.

This book was conceptualized with the vision of imparting up-to-date information and advanced data in this field. To ensure the same, a matchless editorial board was set up. Every individual on the board went through rigorous rounds of assessment to prove their worth. After which they invested a large part of their time researching and compiling the most relevant data for our readers. Conferences and sessions were held from time to time between the editorial board and the contributing authors to present the data in the most comprehensible form. The editorial team has worked tirelessly to provide valuable and valid information to help people across the globe.

Every chapter published in this book has been scrutinized by our experts. Their significance has been extensively debated. The topics covered herein carry significant findings which will fuel the growth of the discipline. They may even be implemented as practical applications or may be referred to as a beginning point for another development. Chapters in this book were first published by InTech; hereby published with permission under the Creative Commons Attribution License or equivalent.

The editorial board has been involved in producing this book since its inception. They have spent rigorous hours researching and exploring the diverse topics which have resulted in the successful publishing of this book. They have passed on their knowledge of decades through this book. To expedite this challenging task, the publisher supported the team at every step. A small team of assistant editors was also appointed to further simplify the editing procedure and attain best results for the readers.

Our editorial team has been hand-picked from every corner of the world. Their multi-ethnicity adds dynamic inputs to the discussions which result in innovative outcomes. These outcomes are then further discussed with the researchers and contributors who give their valuable feedback and opinion regarding the same. The feedback is then collaborated with the researches and they are edited in a comprehensive manner to aid the understanding of the subject.

Apart from the editorial board, the designing team has also invested a significant amount of their time in understanding the subject and creating the most relevant covers. They scrutinized every image to scout for the most suitable representation of the subject and create an appropriate cover for the book.

The publishing team has been involved in this book since its early stages. They were actively engaged in every process, be it collecting the data, connecting with the contributors or procuring relevant information. The team has been an ardent support to the editorial, designing and production team. Their endless efforts to recruit the best for this project, has resulted in the accomplishment of this book. They are a veteran in the field of academics and their pool of knowledge is as vast as their experience in printing. Their expertise and guidance has proved useful at every step. Their uncompromising quality standards have made this book an exceptional effort. Their encouragement from time to time has been an inspiration for everyone.

The publisher and the editorial board hope that this book will prove to be a valuable piece of knowledge for researchers, students, practitioners and scholars across the globe.

List of Contributors

Francis McGlone
School of Natural Sciences and Psychology, Liverpool John Moores University, UK

Robert A. Österbauer
Oxford Centre for Functional Magnetic Resonance Imaging of the Brain, John Radcliffe Hospital, University of Oxford, Oxford, UK

Luisa M. Demattè and Charles Spence
Crossmodal Research Laboratory, Department of Experimental Psychology, University of Oxford, Oxford, UK

Francesco Signorelli
"Magna Græcia" University, Department of Experimental and Clinical Medicine "G. Salvatore", Chair of Neurosurgery, Catanzaro, Italy
Hospices Civils de Lyon, Hôpital Neurologique ET Neurochirurgical, Department of Neurosurgery, Lyon, France

Domenico Chirchiglia
"Magna Græcia" University, Department of Medical and Surgical Sciences, Chair of Neurosurgery, Catanzaro, Italy

Giuseppe Barbagallo
University of Catania, Chair of Neurosurgery, Catania, Italy

Rodolfo Maduri, and Jacques Guyotat
"Magna Græcia" University, Department of Experimental and Clinical Medicine "G. Salvatore", Chair of Neurosurgery, Catanzaro, Italy

Guiomar Niso, Fernando Maestú and Francisco del-Pozo
Center for Biomedical Technology, Technical University of Madrid, Madrid, Spain

Ernesto Pereda
Electrical Engineering and Bioengineering Group, Dept. of Basic Physics, University of La Laguna, Tenerife, Spain

María Gudín and Sira Carrasco
Ciudad Real Universitary Hospital, Ciudad Real, Spain

Jürgen Dammers and Lukas Breuer
Institute of Neuroscience and Medicine, Medical Imaging Physics, INM-4, Forschungszentrum Jülich, Jülich, Germany

Giuseppe Tabbì and Markus Axer
Institute of Neuroscience and Medicine, Structural and Functional Organisation of the Brain, INM-1, Forschungszentrum Jülich, Jülich, Germany

Mirko Avesani and Antonio Fiaschi
University of Verona, Department of Neurological, Neuropsychological, Morphological and Movement Sciences, Italy

Silvia Giacopuzzi
University of Verona, Department of Life and Reproduction Sciences, Italy

Francisco Mercado, Paloma Barjola, Marisa Fernández-Sánchez and Virginia Guerra
Department of Psychology, Faculty of Health Sciences, Rey Juan Carlos University, Madrid, Spain

Francisco Gómez-Esquer
Department of Anatomy and Human Embryology, Faculty of Health Sciences, Rey Juan Carlos University, Madrid, Spain

Teodora-Adriana Perles-Barbacaru and Hana Lahrech
Grenoble Institute of Neurosciences (GIN), French National Institute of Health and Medical Research (INSERM U) – University of Joseph Fourier (UJF) – French Atomic Energy Commission(CEA) – University Hospital of Grenoble (CHU), Bâtiment Edmond J. Safra, Chemin Fortuné Ferrini, La Tronche, France

L. K. Teune, A. L. Bartels and K. L. Leenders
Department of Neurology, University Medical Center Groningen, The Netherlands